The Biology of the Intervertebral Disc

Volume II

Editor

Peter Ghosh, B.SC., Ph.D., A.R.I.C., F.R.A.C.I.
Director
Raymond Purves Research Laboratories at
Royal North Shore Hospital of Sydney
and
Associate Professor,
Department of Surgery
University of Sydney
St. Leonards, N.S.W.
Australia

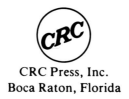

CRC Press, Inc.
Boca Raton, Florida

Library of Congress Cataloging-in-Publication Data

The Biology of the intervertebral disc.

Includes bibliographies and indexes.
1. Intervertebral disk displacement.
2. Intervertebral disk. I. Ghosh, P. (Peter),
1940-   . [DNLM: 1. Intervertebral Disk.
WE 740 B615]
RD771.I6B56   1988   617'.375   87-21781

ISBN 0-8493-6711-5 (v. 1)
ISBN 0-8493-6712-3 (v. 2)

Direct all inquiries to CRC Press, Inc., 2000 Corporate Blvd., N.W., Boca Raton, Florida, 33431.

© 1988 by CRC Press, Inc.

International Standard Book Number 0-8493-6711-5 (v. 1)
International Standard Book Number 0-8493-6712-3 (v. 2)

Library of Congress Card Number 87-21781
Printed in the United States

Dedicated to my wife Nancy, for her support,
encouragement, and understanding during
the difficult times.

FOREWORD

Some long-standing facts, positive recent developments, and certain recent circumstances have set the stage for this timely contribution to the literature. First, one third of all orthopedic referrals are for complaints pertaining to the spinal column. Second, in Western societies, derangements of the intervertebral disc associated with aging, degeneration, and prolapse are the major causes of back pain and allied symptoms. Third, spinal diseases and disorders are the principal cause of physical handicap and activity limitation in the young. In older age groups, they rank third after heart disease and arthritis. Fourth, recent times have seen quantum leaps of knowledge in connective tissue biology — the structure and function of the major macromolecular components collagen(s) and proteoglycan(s), their synthesis and catabolism, and the mechanisms controlling these processes.

Similar (though perhaps less spectacular) advances have been made in ultrastructural research and spinal biomechanics. *Pari passu* with these events has come the clear need for multidisciplinary research. Connective tissues have a "connecting" function which holds implicit connotations for mechanical properties. Now, as perhaps never before, the natural corollaries for connective tissue research are correlative studies. A glance at the cited references in these volumes attests to this.

Nothing is more daunting to a chemist than an uncharacterized mixture, let alone an inability to solubilize its components without their degradation. That, in short, is the situation with which research workers were confronted not so long ago. So the mystery of the collagen molecule could be likened to two equations with three unknowns. The key to proteoglycan structure and its functions started to turn only when it became possible to extract these giant molecules from tissues in their native form, and to purposefully disaggregate them and study their interaction with hyaluronic acid. The technology to unravel the complexities of connective tissue biology is already here, but it would indeed be a great shame if research in molecular biology and applied science in diseases and disorders of the musculoskeletal system became separated. The late Dame Honor Fell often referred to "the unnatural divorce of biochemistry and morphology" and no one attempted reconciliation more than she. Such wise counsel equally applies to biomechanics, morphology, and related areas. To this end, those interested in this "recalcitrant gristle" should take stock of the common clinical problems, where on the basis of existing knowledge, it is reasonable to look towards endeavor in applied research using more than one tool and involving more than one discipline.

To produce this book the editor assembled a group of distinguished scientists, each of whom has made valuable, and original, contributions each in his own field. For this first edition, congratulations are in order. The patent need to assemble such knowledge between the covers of a book assuredly means it will not be the last.

T. K. F. Taylor D.Phil(Oxon), F.R.C.S., F.R.C.S.(Edin), F.R.A.C.S.
Professor of Orthopaedics and Traumatic Surgery
The University of Sydney

PREFACE

While none would deny the importance of the intervertebral disc for normal activity and function, few have earnestly striven to unlock its secrets. The elegant pathoanatomical studies by Püschel, Junghanns, Schmorl, and Hirsch provided early insights into the complexity of this structure, the morphological variations with aging, and frequency of failure in man. Although more than 50 years have elapsed since the observations of Mixter and Barr that disc degeneration and protrusions could be the cause of sciatica, it is only now that some of the enzymes responsible for the turnover of disc matrix components have been identified and a means of their control indicated. It is perhaps because of this paucity of basic knowledge that major advances in the treatment of disc disorders have not been forthcoming. It might be argued by some that chemonucleolysis has provided one solution. However, it must be recognized that we are still uncertain of the manner by which this procedure provides symptomatic relief. Such a situation highlights the need to reappraise the intervertebral disc in the light of our present knowledge and provide new directions for research in the future.

I was therefore delighted to be given the opportunity by CRC Press to bring together the experience and views of some of the leading authorities on disc biology and function in a single treatise. Contributors were selected on the basis of their expertise and were requested to provide an up-to-date review of their area which would be of value to both researchers in the field as well as the uninitiated. The liberal use of prints and line drawings was especially encouraged for we believed that these invarably assist in the interpretation of complex information and ideas. The outcome of this approach has been the production of a two-volume set which covers the disc in terms of its anatomy, growth, assembly, biomechanical function, nutrition, biochemistry, pathology, and response to a variety of therapeutic modalities, including chemonucleolysis. A chapter on the recently developed technique of nuclear magnetic resonance imaging, as applied to the disc, was included because of the strong interest in this subject and its obvious potential for both clinical and research applications.

All contributors were aware of the inadequacies in our knowledge of the disc and were united in their desire to stimulate in others a greater interest in this unique structure. If this review requires revision within the next few years, we will have achieved our objective.

Peter Ghosh
Editor

THE EDITOR

Peter Ghosh, Ph.D. is the Director of the Raymond Purves Research Laboratories at the Royal North Shore Hospital of Sydney, and Associate Professor in the Department of Surgery, the University of Sydney, N.S.W., Australia. Dr Ghosh graduated B.Sc. with Honors from the University of London in 1962. After a year's research in industry, he commenced Ph.D. studies at the University of East Anglia, Norwich, Norfolk, U.K. On Graduating in 1966, Dr. Ghosh was appointed Research Fellow in the Department of Medical Chemistry, John Curtin School of Medical Research, Australian National University, Canberra, A.C.T., Australia. Here he developed strong interests in the mode of action of immunosuppressive and antiinflammatory drugs. This research subsequently led to his appointment to the staff of the Riker Research Institute, Sydney, where he became Head of the Department of Medical Chemistry in 1969. His entry into connective tissue research, particularly the intervertebral disc, commenced in 1971 when he took up the position of National Health and Medical Research Council (NHMRC) Senior Research Officer in the Department of Surgery (Orthopaedic and Traumatic) at the University of Sydney with Professor Thomas Taylor, D.Phil., F.R.C.S. The establishment of Orthopaedic Research Laboratories at the Royal North Shore Hospital of Sydney through a generous donation from the Raymond E. Purves Foundation provided the facilities for an expansion of Dr. Ghosh's activities in connective tissue research and he was appointed as the first Director of the Laboratories in 1973. He was elected Fellow of the Royal Australian Institute of Chemistry in 1975 and awarded the title of Associate Professor, University of Sydney in 1986. He was treasurer of the Connective Tissue Society of Australia and New Zealand from 1976 to 1984 and President from 1984 to 1985. He is a Trustee and scientific advisor to Spinecare, the Children's Spinal Research Foundation, Scientific assessor/advisor for the NHMRC and Medical Research Council of New Zealand, reviewer for *Journal of Rheumatology, Rheumatology International* and *Australian Journal of Biological Sciences,* and consultant for several drug companies. Dr. Ghosh is author or coauthor of 24 book chapters, editorials, review articles, and 125 research publications. He is an active member of several scientific societies including the Orthopaedic Research Society (U.S.), Australian Rheumatism Association, Australian Biochemical Society, Australian Society of Experimental Pathology, and the Australian and New Zealand Society for Cell Biology.

CONTRIBUTORS

Michael A. Adams, Ph.D.
Research Fellow
Department of Anatomy
University of Bristol
Bristol, United Kingdom

Richard M. Aspden, Ph.D.
Research Associate
Department of Medical Biophysics
University of Manchester
Manchester, United Kingdom

Nikolai Bogduk, Ph.D.
Senior Lecturer
Faculty of Medicine
University of Newcastle
Newcastle, Australia

Wallace F. Butler, Ph.D.
Lecturer
Department of Anatomy
School of Veterinary Science
Bristol, United Kingdom

Henry V. Crock, M.D., F.R.A.C.S.
Consultant Spinal Surgeon
Cromwell Hospital
London, England

David R. Eyre, Ph.D.
Ernest M. Burgess Professor of
 Orthopaedic Research
Departments of Orthopaedics and
 Biochemistry
School of Medicine
University of Washington
Seattle, Washington

Peter Ghosh, Ph.D., F.R.A.C.I.
Director
and Associate Professor
Raymond Purves Research Laboratories
The University of Sydney at The Royal
 North Shore Hospital of Sydney
St. Leonards, Australia

Miron Goldwasser, M.D., F.R.A.C.S.
Orthopaedic Surgeon
Sacred Heart Hospital
Coburg, Australia

D. Stephen Hickey, Ph.D.
Research Associate
Department of Medical Biophysics
University of Manchester
Manchester, United Kingdom

David W. L. Hukins, Ph. D.
Senior Lecturer
Department of Medical Biophysics
University of Manchester
Manchester, United Kingdom

William D. Hutton, D. Sc.
Professor
Department of Mechanical Engineering
South Australian Institute of Technology
The Levels, Pooraka
Adelaide, South Australia

Alice Maroudas
Pearl Milch Professor in Biomedical
 Engineering Sciences
Technion-Israel Institute of Technology
Technion City
Haifa, Israel

Cahir A. McDevitt, Ph.D.
Head, Section of Biochemistry
Department of Musculoskeletal Research
The Cleveland Clinic Foundation
 Research Institute
Cleveland, Ohio

James Melrose, Ph.D.
Research Fellow
Raymond Purves Research Laboratories
The University of Sydney at The Royal
 North Shore Hospital of Sydney
St. Leonards, Australia

James R. Taylor, M.D., Ph.D.
Associate Professor
Department of Anatomy and Human
  Biology
The University of Western Australia
Nedlands, Australia

Lance T. Twomey, Ph.D.
Professor and Head
Department of Physiotherapy
Curtin University of Technology
Shenton Park, Australia

**Barrie Vernon-Roberts, M.D., Ph.D.,
  F.R.C.P.A., F.R.C.Path.**
Professor of Pathology
University of Adelaide
Head of Division of Tissue Pathology
Institute of Medical and Veterinary
  Science
Adelaide, Australia

Hidezo Yoshizawa
Professor of Orthopaedic Surgery
Fujita-Gakuen University
School of Medicine
Toyoake, Japan

TABLE OF CONTENTS

Volume 1

Volume 2

Chapter 9

NUTRITION AND METABOLISM OF THE INTERVERTEBRAL DISC

Alice Maroudas

TABLE OF CONTENTS

I. INTRODUCTION

The load-bearing function of the disc depends on the interplay between the two major components of the matrix: collagen and the proteoglycans (PGs). The cells in themselves do not fulfill any direct mechanical function. However, since they need to maintain the matrix throughout life, their role is essential, in particular with respect to the PG turnover. It is therefore obvious that cell nutrition and metabolism are indeed of central importance. The lumbar discs are the largest avascular structures in the body, and it has been suggested that inadequate nutrition and/or accumulation of waste products could be one of the causes of disc degeneration.

In spite of the intrinsic interest of the subject and its possible relevance to back pain, until the 1970s little research had been carried out on transport phenomena in the intervertebral disc. Systematic research in the field had to await the development of suitable in vitro methods.

It must be pointed out in this connection that studying transport phenomena in the disc in vitro is fraught with special difficulties, because the disc swells when placed in contact with solution and tends to lose a major part of its PG. As a result, many of its properties change markedly, and special procedures have to be employed to overcome this.

Disc nutrition depends upon the following factors:

1.   The transport of metabolites to and from the cells through the disc
2.   The area of contact between the avascular disc and the blood vessels at the periphery of the annulus fibrosus and at the bone-disc interface
3.   The rates of consumption and production of various substances by the disc cells

These factors will be discussed in turn.

Since cells in the disc can be as far as 5 to 8 mm from the nearest blood vessel, the transport of metabolites must occur through the matrix of the disc. This transport can occur by molecular diffusion in response to concentration gradients set up during metabolic processes. In addition, solutes are transported by convective flow since they are entrained by the fluid, that is, pumped in and out of the disc during movements accompanying normal activity.

II. PHYSICOCHEMICAL STRUCTURE OF MATRIX

In order to understand the principles governing the two modes of solute transport and to evaluate their relative magnitudes for different types of solutes, it is first necessary to understand certain aspects of the disc's structure from a physicochemical point of view.

The matrix of the disc consists principally of collagen fibers embedded in a gel of PGs and water, the latter containing a number of solutes, both organic and inorganic.

It is the PGs that are responsible for the high water content of the tissue, allied with a low hydraulic permeability and a high swelling pressure. This combination of properties is essential to the load-bearing requirements of the disc.

Since the network formed by the collagen fibrils is much coarser than that due to the PG molecules, it is the proteoglycan-water gel which determines the exclusion volume and the effective pore size of the matrix. Furthermore, after removal of PGs the tissue is uncharged. It is thus the PGs alone that confer a polyelectrolyte behavior on the cartilage matrix.

While the biochemical intricacies of the PG structure are coming increasingly to light (see Chapter 6, Volume I), from the physicochemical point of view the picture is much simpler. Both the osmotic pressure and the pore size of the PG solutions are mainly dependent on the glycosaminoglycan (GAG) component. Thus, it is this component which is the business part of the molecule, the rest being needed mainly for its immobilization within the disc's structure.

A. Matrix Water

Water, containing dissolved solutes, is the main constituent of the disc. Water occupies 65 to 90% of the tissue volume, depending on age and region.[1,2] Since cell density in the disc is very low, most of the water present is extracellular. The water content is determined by the interplay of several factors including the externally applied load, the osmotic pressure of the PG, and the tension in the collagen network.[2-4]

From experiments on solute transport and equilibria in cartilage and the disc, most of the water has been found to be freely exchangeable and fully accessible to small solutes.[1,5-8] However, some of the water is present within the collagen fibrils, while the rest is in the extrafibrillar compartment.[6] In cartilaginous tissues a knowledge of the fraction of intrafibrillar water is of particular importance because, due to their large size, the PGs are excluded from intrafibrillar space. It is, thus, their effective concentration in the *extrafibrillar* space that determines some of the important physicochemical and biomechanical characteristics of cartilage and disc, such as the concentrations of various ions and their rates of penetration, the selective permeability to macromolecular solutes, and the osmotic pressure prevailing in the matrix. The original estimate of intrafibrillar water was 0.7 to 0.8 g/g of collagen for cartilage[10] and 1.33 for the disc nucleus.[11] However, recent studies have shown that the intrafibrillar water is not a constant, but depends on the osmotic pressure prevailing in the extrafibrillar compartment. Thus, the higher the PG concentration in the extrafibrillar matrix, the greater the osmotic activity gradient across the surface of the fibril and the lower the resulting intrafibrillar volume.[11,12]

In a disc of low PG content, high collagen, and low overall hydration, as much as one third to one half of the water in the nucleus under the physiological load would be expected to be intrafibrillar, while in a young nucleus the latter constitutes less than 10% of the total water.[13] Thus, not only is the total water content in an aged disc much lower than in a young disc, but the relative proportion of extrafibrillar water is very much lower still.

The effect of altered hydration on solute transport is complex. On one hand, a decrease in hydration means a lower diffusion coefficient (see Section III.B.1.a), but on the other hand, it means a thinner disc, so that the distances through which metabolites have to travel are smaller. For small solutes, the former effect is of much less significance than the latter as the diffusion coefficients vary relatively little with water content, while the rate of transport is proportional to the square of the distance. A further effect of decreased hydration is the increase in cell density if the overall cell numbers remain the same. This increase would result in an enhanced rate of metabolite consumption and production per unit tissue volume if the rates per cell did not change. The net effect of all these alterations resulting from a decreased water content would be relatively small, because they tend to work in opposite directions and hence to cancel one another out. Thus, decreased hydration as such is not likely to affect significantly the balance between cellular requirements and metabolite transport. However, a decrease in hydration and a parallel thinning of the disc are bound to have an adverse effect on the mechanical properties of the disc itself and, thereby, also on the function of the other components of the spinal segment, in particular on the facet joints.

B. Fixed Charge Density — The Glycosaminoglycans (CS and KS) and Fixed Negative Charge

Chondroitin sulfate (CS) and keratan sulfate (KS) are linear polymers made up of repeating disaccharide units. Their detailed structure is discussed in Chapter 6 (Volume I).

The most important feature of the GAGs is that they are negatively charged. Chondroitin sulfate carries two negative charges per disaccharide (an ester sulfate group on the N-acetyl galactosamine residue and a carboxyl group on the glucuronic acid), while keratan sulfate has one negative charge* per disaccharide (an ester sulfate group on the N-acetyl glucosamine residue).

Thus, the concentration of negatively charged fixed groups is given by the expression

$$FCD = 2CS + KS$$

where FCD is the fixed charge density, CS is the molar concentration of chondroitin sulfate disaccharides, and KS is the molar concentration of keratan sulfate dissacharides.

The above simple relation has been found to hold well in both articular cartilage and the disc.[14-16]

The correspondence between the GAG content and fixed negative charge density makes it possible to use physicochemical methods for the estimation of GAGs, which in many instances are more sensitive and more convenient than the standard biochemical analytical procedures.

Since fixed charge density determines the distribution of ions in the disc, and consequently also their transport, its topographical variations are of considerable importance and will be briefly described. The proportions of the various constituents vary radially across the disc. The composition also varies with age. Typical examples of water content and fixed charge density profiles across L4—L5 discs from individuals of different ages are shown in Figure 1.[13]

Both the water content and the fixed charge density are highest in the nucleus and lowest in the outer annulus. In the older disc the fixed charge density and the hydration are much lower than in the young, and this is particularly noticeable in the nucleus. The older discs exhibit a flatter profile.

It should be noted that, unlike in articular cartilage, the collagen fiber network is rather loose in the disc, especially in the nucleus pulposus. Accordingly, unlike cartilage, the disc tissue can swell, and its water content increases in proportion to its fixed charge density.[17]

C. Partition of Solutes between the Disc and Plasma

Although the major constituent of the disc (and cartilage) matrix is water, the concentration of solutes in this water is not necessarily the same as that in the surrounding plasma. The concentration of solutes in the tissue can be expressed in terms of their concentration in the plasma and a partition coefficient, K. The latter is defined as the ratio of concentration of a given solute in the tissue to that in the plasma when the two phases are in equilibrium.

---

* Although there are indications that KS is often supersulfated, the simple formula only is considered here.

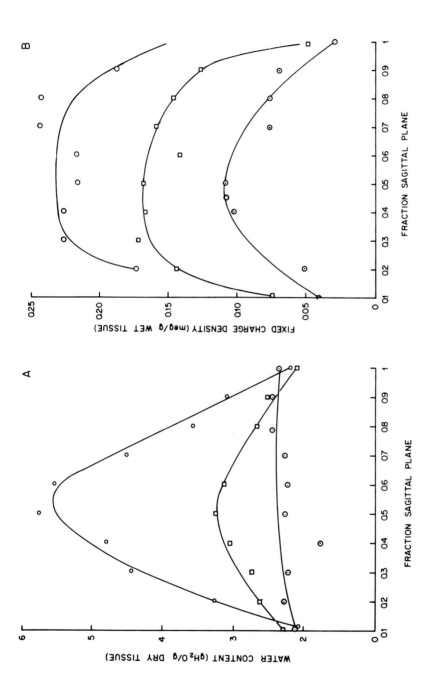

FIGURE 1.   Variations of (A) water content and (B) fixed charge density with position for young and old human L4—L5 lumbar discs. (○, Age 21 years; □, age 60 years; ⊙, age 77 years.)(From Maroudas, A., in preparation.)

1. Ionic Solutes

a. Donnan Equilibrium and Activities

Because of the negatively charged groups immobilized within the matrix, the concentration of mobile ions inside the extracellular fluid is different from that in the plasma. The distribution of the various cations and anions must satisfy two basic conditions: (1) electroneutrality within the tissue, and (2) the equality of the electrochemical potential of each ionic species in the external solution and within the tissue water.[6,18] The above conditions can be expressed by Equations 1 and 2:

$$\overline{m}_x + \Sigma\overline{m}_y = \Sigma\overline{m}_A \tag{1}$$

where $\overline{m}_A$ is the molal concentration of mobile cationic species in the disc water, $\overline{m}_y$ is the molal concentration of mobile anionic species in the disc water, and $\overline{m}_x$ is the molal concentration of negatively charged fixed groups; and

$$\left(\frac{\overline{\alpha}_{cation}}{\alpha_{cation}}\right)^{z\ anion} = \left(\frac{\alpha_{anion}}{\overline{\alpha}_{anion}}\right)^{z\ cation} \tag{2}$$

where $\overline{\alpha}$ is the activity of the given ion in the disc, α is the activity of the given ion in solution, and z is the valency of the ion.

Equation 2 is an expression of the Gibbs-Donnan equilibrium. The activities in Equation 2 can be replaced by the product of molal concentrations and activity coefficients so that

$$\left(\frac{\overline{\gamma}_{cation}\ \overline{m}_{cation}}{\gamma_{cation}\ m_{cation}}\right)^{z\ anion} = \left(\frac{\gamma_{anion}\ m_{anion}}{\overline{\gamma}_{anion}\ \overline{m}_{anion}}\right)^{z\ cation} \tag{3}$$

where $\overline{\gamma}$ and γ are the respective activity coefficients of the ions inside the disc matrix and in solution. If the ionic activities for a given electrolyte are the same inside cartilage as in solution, the electrolyte is said to obey the ideal Donnan equilibrium:

$$\left(\frac{\overline{m}_{cation}}{m_{cation}}\right)^{z\ anion} = \left(\frac{m_{anion}}{\overline{m}_{anion}}\right)^{z\ cation} \tag{4}$$

Thus the activity coefficient ratio $\overline{\gamma}:\gamma$ describes the departure of a given species from its behavior in free solution and is a measure of its interactions with the cartilage matrix. From results on both disc and cartilage as well as, more recently, on PG gels, the activity coefficient ratio for cations as well as for anions has been found to be close to unity. Hence, Equation 4 can be used to describe ionic equilibria between disc tissue and plasma.[1,6,8]

While it is relatively easy to estimate fixed charge density in disc slices, the experimental determination of partition coefficients of ions presents considerable difficulties.[14] Fortunately, in view of the validity of Equations 1 and 4, it is possible to calculate ionic partition coefficients from measured values of fixed charge density. Figure 2 shows the internal concentrations of Na^+ and Cl^- vs. the molal fixed charge density (i.e., the fixed charge density based on total water content) of disc or cartilage in equilibrium with 0.15 MNaCl.[14]

If several different ionic species are present, selectivity coefficients, K_B^A, can be used to describe their relative partitions. In accordance with the Donnan equilibrium, K_B^A is given by the expression

$$K_B^A = (K_A/K_B)^{z_B/z_A} \tag{5}$$

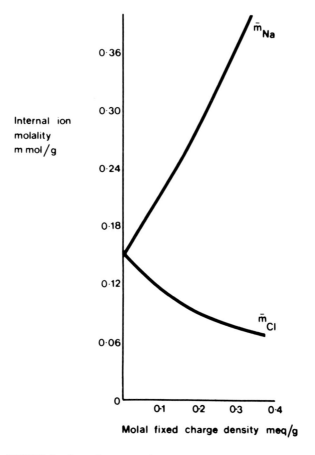

FIGURE 2. Internal concentrations of Na^+ and Cl^- vs. the molal fixed charge density of disc or cartilage in equilibrium with 0.15 MNaCl solution. (From Urban J.P.G. and Maroudas, A., *Biochim. Biophys. Acta*, 586, 166, 1979. With permission.)

where K_A is the partition coefficient of the ion A, K_B is the partition coefficient of the ion B, and the partition coefficient K is defined by $K = \bar{m}/m$. If one ion is present in the external medium at a much lower concentration than another ion, the selectivity coefficient tends to be slightly higher than the value predicted by the Donnan equilibrium equation above. This appears to be the case of the partition coefficient of the sulfate ion at physiological concentrations. Using a value of $K_{Cl^{\pm}}^{SO_4^{2-}} = 1.12^{19}$ and the values of K_{Cl} obtained from Figure 2, the graph of $K_{SO_4^{2-}}$ was obtained as a function of fixed charge density. Because SO_4^{2-} is a divalent ion, its exclusion is greater than that of the univalent Cl^-; hence, its concentration in the tissue is lower. Ionic partition coefficients for Na^+, Cl^-, and SO_4^{2-} calculated from the measured value of fixed charge density for a young and an old disc, respectively, are plotted in Figure 3.

The steep gradients in the measured water content and fixed charge density profiles are reflected in the calculated partition coefficients of the different ions. The concentration of the positively charged Na^+ is highest in the nucleus, where the concentration of PGs (and hence the fixed charge density) is highest. Conversely, the high fixed charge density of the nucleus leads to a strong exclusion of anions. This exclusion is more pronounced for divalent anions such as SO_4^{2-} than for monovalent anions such as Cl^-.

In order to show that the calculated values of the ionic partition coefficients correspond

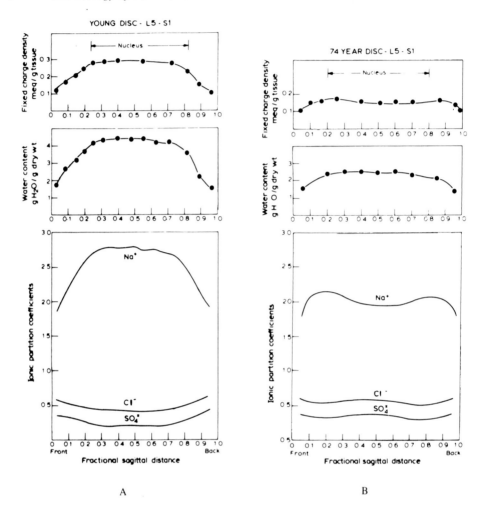

FIGURE 3.   Sagittal profiles of measured fixed charge density and water content, and calculated partition coefficients for Na^+, Cl^-, and SO_4^{2-} across (A) a young (27.4 years) and (B) old (74 years) human L5-S1 disc. (From Urban J.P.G. and Maroudas, A., *Biochim. Biophys. Acta*, 586, 166, 1979. With permission.)

to experimental results, we have plotted in Figure 4 the partition coefficients for SO_4^{2-} determined experimentally for dogs discs. The latter values[7] were obtained by exposing the whole disc to a Ringer's solution containing sodium (^{35}S) sulfate. (It should be noted that, while this would take too long for the human disc, equilibrium can be reached in the smaller canine disc in about 7 days.) The measured values, however, do not reflect those found in vivo because of swelling. The experimental values when plotted against fixed charge density lie very close to the calculated curve, thus justifying the calculation procedure. This agreement also implies that the mean selectivity coefficient for the SO_4^{2-} experimentally determined for human articular cartilage is likely to be the same in the case of the canine intervertebral disc.

The partition coefficient of a solute between the disc matrix and plasma is one of the main factors which determines the rate of transport of that solute. Hence a knowledge of the partition coefficients is very relevant to the description of disc nutrition, and we will return to this topic in Section II.C.2.

b. Internal pH in the Disc Matrix Equation
From the Donnan equilibrium (Equation 1) it follows that the hydrogen ion activity must

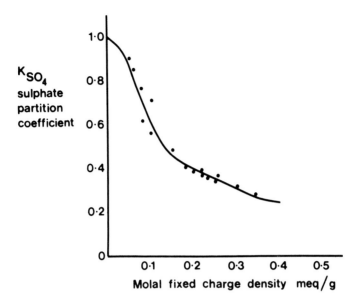

FIGURE 4. Sulfate partition coefficient vs. molal fixed charge density in the intervertebral disc. (—, Calculated curve; •, measured values for dog disc.) (From Urban J.P.G. and Maroudas, A., *Biochim. Biophys. Acta,* 586, 166, 1979. With permission.)

always be higher in the disc than in external solution. The internal pH is given by the formula[6,8]

$$p\overline{H} = pH + \log K_{Cl^-} \tag{6}$$

where pH is the pH of the external solution and K_{Cl^-} is the molal partition coefficient of the chloride ion between disc and external solution.

As we have already seen, the fixed charge density (FCD) in the nucleus of a young disc may reach values around 0.3, with a corresponding K_{Cl^-} of approximately 0.45. Hence,

$$p\overline{H} - pH = -0.35 \tag{7}$$

The internal pH is thus 0.35 units lower than that of the outside solution. The higher the fixed charge density, the lower K_{Cl^-}. Hence, the internal disc pH decreases as the PG concentration increases.

Since PG-degrading enzymes such as cathepsins B and D (see Volume I, Chapter 8) have their optima at acid pH values, the lowering of pH due to the Donnan effect in regions of high fixed charge density, e.g., around cell lacunae, might be of physiological significance.

There is also an additional lowering of pH due to an increased lactic acid concentration in some parts of the tissue, as will be discussed later.

2. Small Uncharged Solutes

Solutes such as urea, glucose, glycine, or proline, which are uncharged at physiological pH and whose dimensions are small compared with the size of the matrix pores, have partition coefficients close to 1.0 in articular cartilage (that is, their concentration in the tissue water — whether extra- or intrafibrillar — is the same as in the external solution).[6,8] In the case of the intervertebral disc, little direct information is available except for some measurements on methyl glucose.[7] Figure 5 shows the variation of the partition coefficient

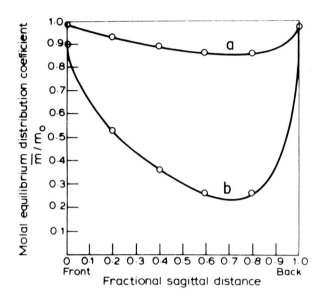

FIGURE 5.   Variations of the partition coefficients of (a) methyl glucose and (b) the sulfate ion as a function of sagittal distance across the disc. (From Holm, S. et al., *Clin. Orthop. Relat. Res.*, 178, 101, 1977. With permission.)

of methyl glucose across a dog's disc as compared with that of the negatively charged sulfate ion. It can be seen that methyl glucose is only minimally excluded from the disk matrix. The slight degree of exclusion (K ~ 0.9), observed within the nucleus where the GAG content is very high, can be attributed to an excluded volume effect.[20] These data are in agreement with the data obtained on glucose in articular cartilage.[6] Hence we may deduce that other small uncharged solutes will also behave similarly.

3. Large Uncharged Solutes

No quantitative information is available on the behavior of large solutes, such as immunoglobulins, in the disc. However, our preliminary results have shown that iodinated serum albumin is excluded form the nucleus. The results of studies on articular cartilage are probably directly applicable to the disc matrix since the exclusion properties are due to the PGs which are present at approximately the same concentrations in both tissues.[6]

Figure 6 gives values of the partition coefficient K, for a range of solutes, as a function of molecular size (Stokes' radius) at one fixed charge density and also shows how K for serum albumin varies with the GAG content (Figure 6B).[22] It can be seen that as the PG content increases, the partition coefficient decreases exponentially. At GAG concentrations corresponding to fixed charge densities greater than 0.15 mEq/mℓ, solutes of the size of serum albumin or larger are virtually excluded from the matrix. Except for the outer region of the annulus fibrosus, the normal disc has a GAG content greater than this.[1,2,13] Therefore, the concentration of large proteins (such as antibodies or certain enzymes) should be negligible in the normal discs. However, degenerate discs, where the PG content of the nucleus is lowered, could allow greater access to degradative enzymes, thus accelerating tissue destruction.

Another practical point of interest should be mentioned in this connection. One of the methods of assessing the integrity of the disc is the so-called discography, which consists in injecting a solution of a large molecule labeled with iodine into the disc and following its path on X-ray. We believe that the path of the macromolecule is along a *defect* in the

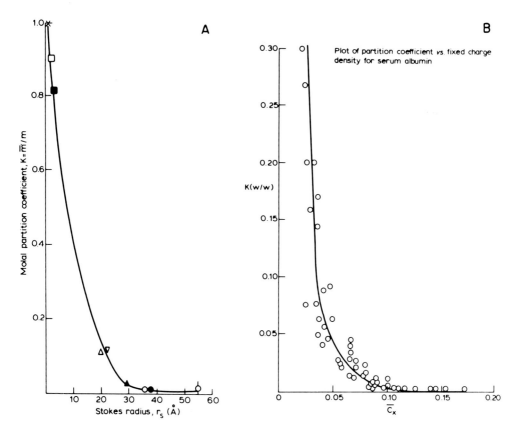

FIGURE 6.   (A) Variations in the molal partition coefficient with solute size. (×, Urea and proline; □, glucose; ■, sucrose; △, myoglobin; ▽, chymotrypsinogen; ▲, ovalbumin; ○, serum albumin; ●, transferrin; ⌀ , IgG.) (From Maroudas, A., *J. Anat.,* 120, 335, 1976. With permission.) (B) Variations in the partition coefficient of serum albumin, K (w/w), with the glycosaminoglycan content, $\overline{C}$x. $\overline{C}$x is in millimoles per gram of tissue. (From Maroudas, A., in *Adult Articular Cartilage,* 2nd ed., Freeman, M. A. R., Ed., Pitman Medical, London, 1973. With permission.)

disc structure and not through the matrix itself since the macromolecule must be excluded from the matrix.

III. TRANSPORT THROUGH THE MATRIX

A. General Principles

Having described the physicochemical structure of the matrix, we will now consider the mechanisms of transport through that matrix.

Solutes move through the matrix disc under concentration gradients set up between the avascular supply and the discs' cells. The distances for diffusion are large. In adult human discs, some cells may be as much as 5 to 8 mm from the blood supply, since a human lumbar disc is typically about 10 to 16 mm thick and 30 mm across its shortest diameter. Solute transport may also be assisted by fluid flow, as solutes are entrained in the fluid which is pumped in and out of the disc under changing loads. Mathematically, the rate of solute transport can be expressed in the following form:[18]

$$J = -\left(\overline{D}\, \frac{d\overline{C}}{dx} + \overline{C} \cdot \kappa\, \frac{dp}{dx} \right) \tag{8}$$

where J is the total solute flux mol/sec/cm, D is the diffusion coefficient of the solute inside the disc, $\overline{C}$ is the equilibrium solute concentration in the disc, $d\overline{C}/dx$ is the concentration gradient of the solute in the disc, κ is the hydraulic permeability coefficient, and dp/dx is the hydrostatic pressure gradient.

Strictly, for diffusion of electrolytes, a further term needs to be added, diffusive transport, being given by the Nernst-Planck equation:[18]

$$ J_{diff} = -\overline{D}_i \left(\frac{d\overline{C}_i}{dx} + z_i \overline{C}_i \frac{F}{RT} \frac{d\phi}{dx} \right) \tag{9} $$

where i is any of the mobile species present, F is the Faraday constant, and $d\phi/dx$ is the electric potential gradient. If an ion is present in very small quantities, the second term in Equation 9 becomes negligible. This condition applies, for instance, to the flux of the sulfate ion within cartilage or the disc since its concentration is of the order of 0.4 mM.

B. Diffusion Coefficients
1. Small Solutes
a. In Vitro Measurements

The diffusion coefficient D characterizes the rate at which a solute moves by molecular diffusion: the larger the value of D, the faster the rate of diffusion. D varies considerably with the size of the solute: in aqueous solution the diffusion coefficient of the small chloride ion is 20.4×10^{-6} cm²/sec at 25°C,[21] while that of serum albumin is 6.4×10^{-7} cm²/sec at 25°C,[22] i.e., 30 times smaller.

Solutes diffuse more slowly in the disc than in free solution. This is due to the presence of solids within the tissue which act as obstacles and lead to an increased tortuosity; the solute has to move through a longer path to cover a given distance than it would in free solution.

The difficulty of measuring the diffusion coefficients in the disc arises from the fact that both steady state techniques (i.e., those involving a diffusion cell) and desorption techniques, such as have been used for articular cartilage,[5,22] involve contact between tissue and solution, and under these conditions disc slices swell very quickly and lose PGs. Consequently, a different system was used which avoids contact between the tissue and external solution.[1]

The principle of the method is as follows. A spot of radioactive tracer is placed at one end of a thin strip of disc at the time t = 0. The tracer diffuses through the strip, the tracer molecules interchanging with the solute molecules. The driving force for diffusion is the specific activity gradient. A concentration profile of radioactive tracer develops through the slice. By analyzing this profile at a known time t, the tracer diffusion coefficient in the tissue $\overline{D}$ can be obtained.

Using the above procedure, the diffusion coefficients given in Table 1 were obtained by Urban[1] for a number of solutes. The experimental values were based on the tissue water content and were obtained at 4°C. They were converted to a whole tissue basis using the relation $\overline{D}_{water} = \overline{D}_{tissue}/\epsilon^2$, where ϵ is the volume fraction of water in the tissue. The values at 25°C were calculated from those at 4°C using the following equation:[23]

$$ \ln \overline{D}_{25°C} = \ln \overline{D}_{4°C} + \frac{E}{R} \left(\frac{1}{227} - \frac{1}{298} \right) \tag{10} $$

where E is the activation energy (4 kcal).

It can be seen from Table 1 that the ratio $\overline{D}_{water}/D$ is similar for all the solutes tested, whether uncharged (tritiated water, THO), cationic (Na^+, Ca^{2+}), or anionic (Cl^- and SO_4^{2-}). The mean value of this ratio is

Table 1
DIFFUSION COEFFICIENTS OF SOME SOLUTES IN
THE DISC COMPARED WITH VALUES IN FREE
SOLUTION

	$\overline{D}_{water} \times 10^6$		$D \times 10^6$ cm²/sec	$\overline{D}_{water} / D$
Solute	4°C (measured)	25°C (calculated)	25°C	25°C
Na⁺	5.18	8.6	13.3[47]	0.64
Cl⁻	8.06	13.5	20.4[47]	0.66
SO₄²⁻	2.16	3.6	6.3[48]	0.58
Ca²⁺	3.02	5.0	7.9[47]	0.63
HTO	10.8 (8°C)	15.4	22.6[47]	0.63

Note: $\overline{D}_{water}$, diffusivity in the disc based on water content; D, diffusivity in aqueous solution; HTO, tritiated water.

$$\frac{\overline{D}_{water}}{D} = 0.63 \tag{11}$$

Hence, from Equations 10 and 11 it follows that

$$\frac{\overline{D}_{tissue}}{D} = 0.63 \ \epsilon^2 \tag{12}$$

The fact that there was no retardation of Na⁺ or Ca²⁺ relative to THO or Cl⁻ showed that under physiological conditions the cations were in no way bound or localized by the negatively charged groups. This was consistent with the experimental results reported for cartilage as well as with the recent experiments and theoretical considerations applying to chondroitin sulfate and hyaluronic acid-water gels.[24]

The reduction in the diffusion coefficient in the disc as compared with free solution can be explained in terms of a reduction in the effective area available to the diffusing molecules and an increase in the tortuosity of the path due to the solids present in the tissue. A formula derived by Mackie and Meares[25] for porous media and based purely on geometrical considerations relates $\overline{D}_{tissue}$ to D as follows:

$$\frac{\overline{D}_{tissue}}{D} = \frac{\epsilon^2}{(2 - \epsilon)^2} \tag{13}$$

With ϵ varying from 0.6 to 0.85 (i.e., for water contents from 50 to 80% by weight), Equations 12 and 13 give similar reductions in the diffusion coefficient $\overline{D}_{tissue}$ compared with D. At a water content of 70% (grams of H_2O per gram of dry tissue = 2.33; ϵ = 0.77) both equations give the same value of $\overline{D}/D$:0.4. At 80% H_2O (grams of H_2O per gram of dry tissue = 4; ϵ = 0.85) Equation 12 yields $\overline{D}/D$ = 0.46, while Equation 13 gives $\overline{D}/D$ = 0.54. At 50 % H_2O (grams of H_2O per gram of dry tissue = 1; ϵ = 0.59) Equation 12 gives $\overline{D}/D$ = 0.37, and Equation 13 gives $\overline{D}/D$ = 0.3.

Thus, even at the extreme ends of the physiological range it appears that the reduction of the diffusion coefficient can be estimated reasonably well from an equation based purely on considerations of increased tortuosity and reduction in free cross-sectional area within the tissue matrix.

Apart from the results given in Table 1 due to Urban,[1] two other sources of information relating to solute diffusion in the disc exist. Paulson and Sylven[26] measured $\overline{D}/D$ for a range of solutes in the nucleus pulposus using a method similar to that described above. The average water content of their samples was 84%, and they found $\overline{D}/D$ for nonelectrolytes to be about 0.5, which agrees with the predictions based on Equation 12 above. The other measurements were due to Nachemson et al.,[27] who obtained the diffusion coefficient of glucose in the outer annulus using a diffusion cell; the value of $\overline{D}/D$ was about 0.4, again in agreement with Equation 12.

It is thus clear that the values of the diffusion coefficient in the intervertebral disc at a given water content can be predicted, with reasonable accuracy, using either Equation 12 based on empirical results or the more fundamental Equation 13.

Furthermore, it can be concluded that the values of the diffusion coefficient in the disc are similar to those in articular cartilage of the same water content.

The variations in the values of the diffusion coefficient with hydration within the physiological hydration range are not very large and are not expected to play a major role in determining changes in nutrient supply to the cells (see Section II.A).

b. In Vivo Measurements

Because the articular cartilage of most experimental animals is very thin, any tracer injected intravenously very rapidly reaches an equilibrium concentration in cartilage. It is therefore difficult to test the accuracy of the diffusion equation in vivo for this tissue. However, it is possible to do so for the intervertebral disc, which has very much larger dimensions. There are two routes for the transport of solutes into the disc: from the peripheral vessels into the annulus fibrosus and via the central portion of the end-plate into the nucleus (for further details see Section IV.A). If tracer is introduced intravenously into dogs which are sacrificed at different time intervals after the injection, it is possible to measure the concentration of tracer as a function of position within the disc and of time. The profiles thus obtained can be compared with those predicted by the use of diffusion equations provided the diffusion and partition coefficients of the given solute are known.[7]

Figure 7A shows graphs of inorganic (^{35}S) sulfate distribution as a function of distance across the disc.[28] The theoretical curves were calculated from equations based on Fick's law, using the diffusion coefficient and the partition data obtained from in vitro studies and assuming diffusion from the periphery only. The measured level of inorganic (^{35}S) sulfate follows the calculated curve closely in the outer annulus, and the two diverge only where the diffusion from the end-plate makes its additional contribution.[7,28]

The above agreement between theory and experimental results is very important as it clearly demonstrates that the diffusion coefficients measured in vitro can be used to describe solute transport in vivo and to predict it under various conditions.

2. Higher-Molecular-Weight Solutes

The mobility of molecules decreases with their size. Hence, the diffusion coefficients in aqueous solution of solutes such as serum albumin or IgG are much lower than those of small solutes. Thus, for instance, $D_{albumin}$ is an order of magnitude lower than $D_{glucose}$.[8] Moreover, for molecules whose dimensions are not negligible in relation to pore size, the diffusion coefficients depend, not only on the friction between the solute and the solvent, but also on the friction between the solute molecules and the solid elements in the matrix. Hence Equation 12 or 13 will no longer hold. Corrections for size effects have been attempted.

Faxen,[29] for instance, calculated the reduction in mobility of a spherical particle in a cylindrical pore by friction with the pore walls.

Ogston et al.,[30] on the basis of a stochastic model, suggested the following relation between $\overline{D}$ and D for compact molecules in solution of chain polymers:

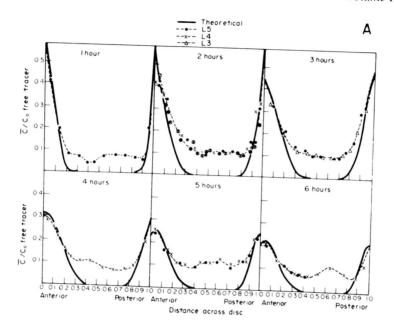

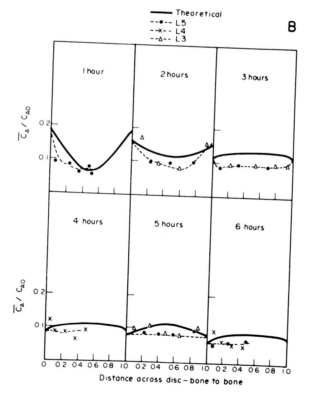

FIGURE 7.   Free (^{35}S) sulfate concentration profile at 1 to 6 hr after injection. (A) Sagittal section across canine disc. (B) Bone-to-bone section through the nucleus. (——, Calculated curve for diffusion from the annulus edge; - - - , experimental curve.) (From Urban, J.P.G. et al., *Biorheology*, 15, 203, 1978. With permission.)

$$\frac{\overline{D}}{D} = \exp(-B\sqrt{C_x}) \tag{14}$$

where C_x is the concentration of chain polymers and B is a function of the solute radius r_s.

No direct measurements of the diffusion coefficients of large solutes in the disc have been made. However, data obtained on articular cartilage give ratios of $\overline{D}$:D of around 0.25 to 0.3,[8] which is more or less consistent with Equation 14.

The overall rate of diffusion of large globular proteins into tissues, such as cartilage or disc, is very low due to the low value of both the partition coefficients and the diffusion coefficients. Thus, there should be practically no penetration of large molecules (e.g., proteins) into nondegenerate, young discs having a high PG content and no fissures.

IV. PERMEABILITY OF THE DISC INTERFACE

In life, solutes have to be transported to and from the avascular disc by the blood vessels surrounding the disc. It has been known for a number of years that nutrition of articular cartilage takes place mainly through the articular surface, the bone interface being almost impermeable. However, the intervertebral disc is a much larger avascular structure, and solute supply from the periphery of the annulus alone could not be sufficient to provide nutrients to the cells in the nucleus. Thus, *a priori* it was to be expected that there should be a more direct route to the nucleus.

A. Routes of Supply

Early qualitative work indeed showed that the latter was the case. Thus, Brodin,[31] by injecting a fluorescent dye into rabbits, found that penetration into the disc occurred from the edge of the annulus and also, but to a smaller extent, from the vertebral bodies through the end-plates.

A qualitative in vitro investigation of the adult human intervertebral disc[32] showed that the calcified zone of the end-plate is partly permeable to solutes, this being associated with the presence of vascular contacts between the marrow spaces of the vertebral body and the hyaline cartilage of the end-plate. The central portion of the end-plate was found to be more permeable than the rest, the degree of permeability varying widely among individuals. The annulus was always permeable. The above studies thus indicated that the possible routes for the nutrition of the disc are through the annulus from the surrounding blood vessels and through the end-plates. However, it was not possible to assess from those qualitative results the relative importance of the two routes.

B. Quantitation of the Supply Routes: In Vivo Studies in the Dog

The relative contribution of the two routes was subsequently quantified in an in vivo study on adult dogs.[7,28] In this study, radioactively labeled (^{35}S) sulfate and (^{3}H) methyl glucose solutions were injected intravenously into a number of dogs. Tracer profiles were obtained in the disc after the dogs had been killed, following different time intervals. The decay of radioactivity from blood plasma was simultaneously monitored so that the radioactivity in the tissue could be normalized. From a knowledge of the partition and diffusion coefficients of the solutes employed, it was possible to predict the profiles of tracer-labeled sulfate and methyl glucose on the basis of the following assumptions:

1.   The outer surface of the disc is in tracer equilibrium with the plasma. (Experimental results have shown this to be the case.)
2.   The tracer distributes itself between the plasma and tissue as predicted from in vitro experiments. The rate of consumption of the tracer by the cells is nil in the case of

methyl glucose and negligible within the experimental time in the case of (^{35}S) sulfate.

3. Since it is known that transport into the disc is by two distinct routes, i.e., through the periphery of the annulus and through the central portion of the end-plate,[7,28] and since, under the experimental conditions used, the time for tracer diffusion was short compared to the size of the discs, it was possible to make the approximation that the two routes are independent of each other. Transport could thus be described by one-dimensional equations.[7]

Figure 7 shows both the calculated and the experimental profiles for the (^{35}S) sulfate from 1 to 6 hr after injection. In Figure 7A the sagittal section is shown, while in Figure 7B the bone-bone profile is given for the region of the nucleus.

It can be seen from Figure 7B that the actual results lie only 10 to 20% lower than the theoretical, which implies that most of the bone-disc interface must be permeable. The small discrepancy is likely to be due, at least in part, to the fact that some radial diffusion is probably also occurring.

By calculating the theoretical flux for the inner annulus, it was found that because the mean partition coefficient in this region is almost double that in the nucleus, the flux should be double as well. In fact, the experimental value of the flux was either equal to or lower than that in the region of the nucleus (Figure 7A). Calculations based on the mean value of the flux showed that about 35% of the bone-disc interface in the region of the inner annulus is permeable. In the outer annulus, since the experimental points coincide with the curve predicted for diffusion from periphery only, diffusion via the end-plate must be negligible.

On an overall basis, if one calculates the total theoretical flux from the end-plate, taking into account the appropriate partition coefficients for the different regions, one gets a value which is equal to more than twice the value obtained experimentally. Thus, only about 40% of the bone-disc interface is permeable, the most permeable region being the nucleus and the least being the outer annulus.

The experimental curve for the uncharged methyl glucose is given in Figure 8 for a time interval of 2 hr. It is rather different from that for the sulfate ion because here there is very little solute exclusion in the region of the nucleus. The amount of tracer supplied via the end-plate is, in this case, much larger than before. It is not possible by this treatment to calculate precisely the relative contributions of the two routes because, due to considerable radial diffusion from the nucleus to the annulus, they are no longer independent, and the one-dimensional theoretical treatment breaks down.

For an uncharged solute such as methyl glucose, if the same fraction of the end-plate is as permeable as for the sulfate ion, the approximate contribution per unit cross-sectional area of the end-plate will be equal to 40% of that per unit cross-sectional area of the annulus. Since in the dog's disc the total bone-disc interface is approximately twice as large as the periphery of the annulus, the permeable area of both end-plates together works out to be more or less equal to that of the periphery. Figure 9 shows the variation in the permeable fraction of the bone-disc interface across the disc. The values calculated for the different regions agree approximately with the visual evidence of blood vessel contact (Figure 10).

Although the permeable area is clearly the same for all solutes, the relative proportion of a particular solute that will diffuse via each route will depend on the distribution coefficient of that solute at each interface and hence on the GAG (or fixed charge density) profile across the disc. As we have seen for a small anion such as sulfate, the amount supplied through the periphery of the annulus is almost twice as much as that diffusing through the end-plates. For a small, uncharged solute such as glucose, the two routes will be of equal importance, but for cations it is the end-plate route that will be the more effective.

It is obvious that while some of the conclusions obtained in the above studies can be directly extrapolated to the human disc, the questions as to the exact fraction of the bone/

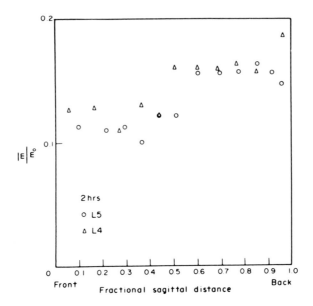

FIGURE 8.   Variations of tracer methyl glucose concentration across the disc at 2 hr after injection.($\bigcirc$ L5 disc. $\triangle$ L4 disc.) (From Urban, J.P.G. et al., *Biorheology*, 15, 203, 1978. With permission.)

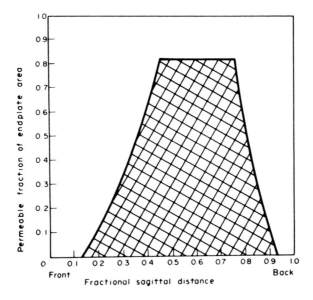

FIGURE 9.   Sketch of the permeable fraction of the end-plate across a sagittal section of dog disc. (From Urban, J.P.G. et al., *Biorheology*, 15, 203, 1978. With permission.)

end-plate interface which is permeable to solutes in man and whether this is constant or varies from individual to individual have not, up to the present, even been approached. If one is to judge the nutritional status of human discs in relation to the metabolic requirements, in vitro methods have to be developed to quantify the permeability of the bone-disc interface in human individuals.

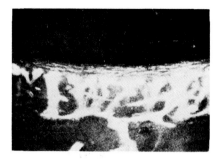

A

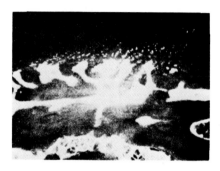

B

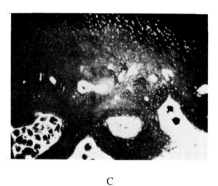

C

FIGURE 10. Photographs of blood vessels at the bone-disc interface in the region of (A) nucleus pulposus, (B) mid-zone of annulus fibrosus, and (C) outer annulus fibrosus. (From Urban, J.P.G. et al., *Biorheology*, 15, 203, 1978. With permission.)

V. DOES PUMPING CONTRIBUTE TO THE NUTRITION OF THE INTERVERTEBRAL DISC?

Because of the large distances for solute transport in the avascular disc, it has been suggested that convective solute transport is necessary for its nourishment. However, the disc matrix offers a high resistance to fluid flow[1,4,33] and therefore has a low hydraulic permeability.

In order to assess quantitatively the contribution of fluid flow to the overall transport, the mechanisms of fluid flow during load bearing have to be considered in some detail.[1,33,34]

A. Mechanisms of Fluid Flow Accompanying Load Bearing

In man, the intervertebral disc is always under load. The load arises partly from body weight and partly from muscle and ligament tension. It is very dependent on posture. Nachemson and Elfstrom[35] found that even in supine subjects intradiscal pressure in the L3 disc was 0.1 to 0.2 MPa, corresponding to a load of about 250 N, whereas in the same subject in unsupported sitting the pressure was about 0.6 to 0.7 MPa, corresponding to about 700 N. Postures involving flexion and extension increase the pressure within the disc considerably. During strenuous activity, peak intradiscal pressures can rise to over 1.6 MPa.[36,37] Because of the relationship between disc pressure and posture in humans, the load on the spine tends to follow a cyclic pattern. It is at its lowest during rest at night and then increases during the day's activities. The alterations in pressure significantly affect the height of the disc. If a load is suddenly applied, the deformation arises initially mainly from a rearrangement of the collagen network.[38] However, if the increased load is maintained, the disc creeps, and its volume changes slowly as fluid is squeezed out (and with it possibly some solutes). At equilibrium, when there is no net fluid loss or gain from the disc, its swelling pressure P_{S_1} exactly balances the applied pressure P_{A_1}:

$$P_{A_1} = P_{S_1} \tag{15}$$

The net swelling pressure (P_S) of a disc (or cartilage) results from the difference between the swelling tendency of the PGs due to their osmotic pressure, π, and the resisting forces of the collagen network, P_C:

$$P_S = \pi - P_C \tag{16}$$

P_S is determined by measuring the applied pressure, P_A, which is required to stop the tissue from gaining or losing water. For a given tissue specimen, it varies with the extent of hydration.

The osmotic pressure of the PGs, π, consists of two components, which are simply additive.[39] These components are the Donnan swelling pressure, P_{Don}, which results from the excess of positive counterions in the tissue due to the polyanionic nature of the GAGs, and P_{excl}, which is an entropic contribution resulting from the steric exclusion which the polymer chains exert upon one another.

$$\pi = P_{Don} + P_{excl} \tag{17}$$

Both components depend on GAG concentration. However, at concentrations of GAGs present in cartilaginous tissues P_{Don} is the dominant term, being responsible for three fourths of the total osmotic pressure developed by the PGs.[39]

In order to estimate the effective osmotic pressure of the PGs in a piece of tissue from a knowledge of the osmotic pressure of the pure PG, it is not sufficient to know the overall PG content of the tissue specimen, but it is necessary to know the actual PG concentration based on the extrafibrillar water.

In view of the dependence of P_S on the PG concentration, it is not surprising to find a decrease in P_S with age and, hence, a lower disc hydration under a given applied pressure in an aged as compared with a young subject (Figure 11).

So far, we have only considered the conditions which determine the hydration of a disc at equilibrium. Let us now examine the dynamics of fluid flow accompanying load bearing.

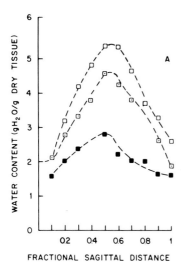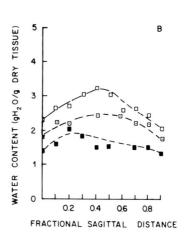

FIGURE 11. Sagittal profiles of measured water content for L4-L5 discs from (A) a 17-year-old and (B) a 60-year-old individual at different applied pressures. (□, as cut; ▪, at 2 atm applied pressure; ■, at 5 to 8 atm applied pressure.) (From Ziv, I. and Maroudas, A., in preparation.)

If the applied load is increased so that $P_{A_2} > P_{A_1}$, the disc is no longer at equilibrium. Since $P_{A_2} > P_{S_1}$, fluid is squeezed out of the disc. As fluid is lost, the concentration of the PGs increases, and consequently their osmotic pressure rises. At the same time, as the volume of the disc decreases through loss of fluid, the collagen network tension decreases. Both these changes tend to increase the disc's swelling pressure, P_S. Flow continues until the net pressure applied to the disc equals the increased swelling pressure.

Virtually all treatments of flow through connective tissue, including disc, use models in which tissues contain interconnecting water-filled pores through which fluid flow takes place. The flow is assumed to follow Darcy's law, i.e.,

$$q = -kA \frac{dP}{dx} \tag{18}$$

where q is the flow rate, k is the hydraulic permeability, A is the cross-sectional area of the tissue, and dP/dx is the pressure gradient across the segment.

During the process of tissue compression (i.e., during creep) the driving force for fluid outflow is the difference between the externally applied pressure, P_A, and the tissue swelling pressure, P_S.[3,8]

The equation for fluid flow has to be rewritten in the form

$$q = -A\kappa(H) \frac{d[P_a - P_S(H)]}{dx} \tag{19}$$

where both κ and P_S are functions of the water content, H. During fluid imbibition, accompanying tissue relaxation, the driving force for fluid flow into the tissue is provided by net swelling pressure.

Using the above concepts and the continuity equation for fluid flow, Fatt and Goldstick[40] derived an equation for estimating fluid flow in the cornea, which is analogous in the form to the diffusion equation. This equation, slightly modified, has been successfully used to describe fluid flow in the disc.[33] The equation is

$$\frac{\partial H}{\partial t} = \frac{\partial}{\partial z} \left[D(H) \frac{dH}{dz} \right] \tag{20}$$

where H is hydration; t is time; z is the distance based on dry tissue volume; and D(H) is the water transport coefficient, analogous to a concentration-dependent diffusion coefficient, since it is a function of water content. It is defined by the expression

$$D(H) = \kappa \frac{V_s}{(V_s + H)} \frac{dP}{dH} \tag{21}$$

where κ is the hydraulic permeability coefficient; V_s is the specific volume of the dry disc material; and dP is the pressure gradient causing flow, which by Starling's hypothesis depends on both hydrostatic and osmotic pressure differences between intradiscal fluid and fluid within the surrounding unstressed tissue. D(H) and κ depend on H (Figure 12), and hence both depend on PG content.

By defining a mean transport coefficient D(H) over a hydration range and determining it under given physiological conditions, its value can be compared to that of the diffusion coefficient, and this will yield a measure of the relative contributions of fluid flow and molecular diffusion to the transport of various solutes. Since the diffusivities of common small solutes range between 3×10^{-6} and 6×10^{-6} cm²/sec, whereas the transport coefficients range between 2×10^{-8} and 2×10^{-7} cm²/sec, it follows that the contribution of fluid flow will be one to two orders of magnitude less than that of molecular diffusion.

On the other hand, as far as larger solutes (such as serum albumin) are concerned, the diffusion coefficients are of the order of 10^{-7} cm²/sec[22], i.e., of about the same order of magnitude as the transport coefficient $\overline{D}(H)$. Thus, in the case of the larger solutes, fluid flow may play an important part in their transport through the matrix.

B. In Vivo Experiments

In order to assess experimentally in vivo if there is any observable contribution of motion to the transport of small solutes, the series of experiments described in Section III.B.1.b with anesthetized dogs was repeated on dogs which were made to run during the whole duration of the experiment.[41]

If fluid flow had significantly affected the rate of transport, the measured experimental profiles should have diverged from the calculated curves, at least in the latter case. However, there was no significant difference between the measured and the calculated profiles in either case (Figure 13).

Although the load distribution is clearly different in dogs and humans, the stresses on the dog's spine must be larger during load bearing and exercise than when the dogs are lying anesthetized. The fact that no difference in the distribution of radioactively labeled sulfate was observed between the two groups of dogs implies that load bearing, and hence the fluid flow, has little effect on intradiscal transport of a small solute such as the sulfate ion, which agrees with our theoretical calculations.

VI. CELL METABOLISM AND MATRIX TURNOVER

A. Cell Density

The cell density of the disc is low, much lower even than in articular cartilage, which is well in keeping with the long distances between some regions of the disc and the nearest blood vessels. Cell concentration is highest near the end-plate and at the periphery of the annulus, that is, close to the routes of nutrient supply (Figure 14).[42]

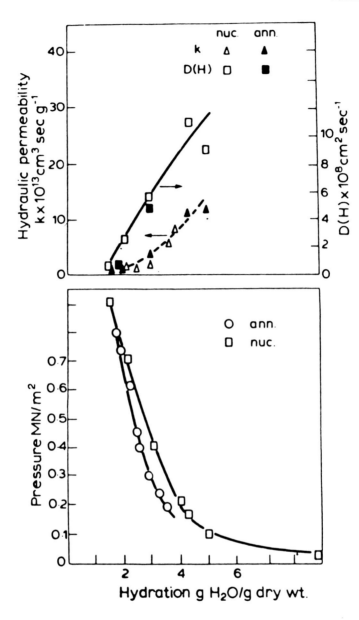

FIGURE 12. Dependence of hydraulic permeability (h) and transport coefficient D(H) on tissue hydration. (From Urban, J. and Maroudas, A., in *Engineering Aspects of the Spine,* Institution of Mechanical Engineers Publications, London, 1980. With permission.)

Table 2 gives a comparison of cell densities in different regions of the human and the canine discs. It should be pointed out that the cell density data on the human disc are probably an underestimate because it has been found that even whole discs swell during fixation.[43]

B. Proteoglycan Production and Turnover

Apart from the intrinsic interest attached to the rates of synthesis of PGs in tissues, the question of how rapidly the PGs can be replaced is central to the problem of the likelihood of matrix repair in pathological states such as disc degeneration, which are known to be characterized by a decrease in the PG content of the tissues involved.

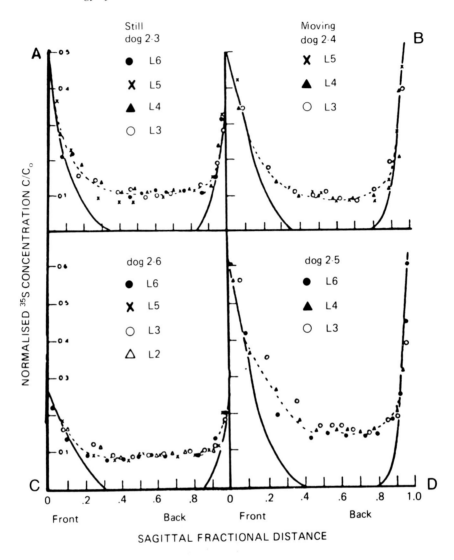

FIGURE 13.   Normalized (^{35}S) sulfate profile across discs of dogs killed 2 hr after tracer injection: sagittal section. (A, C) Anesthetized dogs; (B, D) moving dogs. (——, Calculated curve for diffusion from annulus periphery; - - -, curve through experimental points; L2—6 represent intervertebral discs in the lumbar region of the spine.) (From Urban, J. P. G. et al., *Clin. Orthop. Relat. Res.,* 170, 209, 1982. With permission.)

One of the easiest methods of assessing the rate of PG synthesis is from measurements of sulfate incorporation into the GAG.

1. Principles Underlying the Determination of Sulfate Metabolism from Tracer Incorporation
    The principle of the method for determining the rate of sulfate uptake (or that of any other precursor) from tracer incorporation, whether carried out in vivo or in vitro, is as follows.[44] The radioactive tracer which has been introduced into the incubation medium (in the case of in vitro work) or into the animal's bloodstream (in an in vivo experiment) diffuses into the aqueous phase of the disc and is thence taken up by the cells, is incorporated into the newly synthesized structural molecules, and becomes fixed within the matrix. In order to obtain the incorporation rate, the mean radioactivity due to the free tracer in the tissue

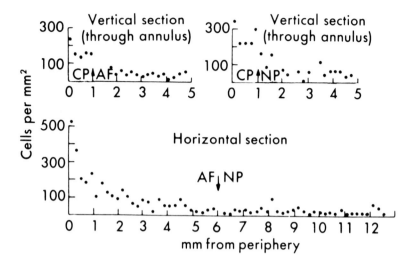

FIGURE 14. Distribution of cells in the intervertebral disc of an 18-year-old. (CP, cartilage end-plate; AF, annulus fibrosus; NP, nucleus pulposus; arrows indicate transitions.) (From Maroudas, A. et al., *J. Anat.*, 120, 113, 1975. With permission.)

Table 2
SUMMARY OF OXYGEN CONSUMPTION RATES AND CELL DENSITIES FOR SOME AVASCULAR TISSUE, INCLUDING TWO VASCULARIZED TISSUES FOR COMPARISON

Tissue	Oxygen consumption rate (Q; μmol O_2/g/hr)	Cell density (cells/mm³ × 10^{-3})	Oxygen respiration (μmol O_2/cell/hr)
Cartilage			
Rat	8.93—2.95	250	0.39—0.13
Rabbit	4.46	250	0.20
	2.01	128	0.16
	2.14—0.89	250	0.09—0.04
Dog	0.59	39.5	0.17
Young bovine	1.16	133.0	0.088
Adult bovine	0.31	47.2	0.068
Old bovine	0.11	34.0	0.032
Disc			
Inner annulus, human	0.076[a]	5.0	0.16
Nucleus, human	0.063[a]	4.3	0.16
Inner annulus, dog	0.25	16.1	0.16
Liver, rabbit	344	620	5.54
Kidney, rabbit	484	1100	4.38

[a]   Calculated by extrapolation from the respiration data.

(i.e., the tracer within the aqueous phase of the matrix) must be determined separately from that due to the tracer incorporated into the structural molecules. Provided the concentration of the free sulfate ion in the matrix is known, it is possible, from a simple mass balance, to calculate the rate, Q, of sulfate uptake into the GAGs. Thus, Q is given by

$$Q = \frac{N_{inc} \times \overline{C}_{free}}{N_{free} \times t} \qquad (22)$$

where N_{inc} is the detected radioactivity due to ^{35}S present as incorporated sulfate per gram of wet tissue, N_{free} is the detected radioactivity due to ^{35}S present as free inorganic sulfate per gram of tissue (mean value over the duration of the experiments), and $\overline{C}_{free}$ is the steady state concentration of free sulfate in the tissue in millimoles per gram of tissue.

Unfortunately, $\overline{C}_{free}$ is not usually measurable in the disc as it is very small compared with the organic sulfate. If the rate of consumption for the free sulfate is low compared with its rate of diffusion into the tissue, its concentration can be obtained from the value of the equilibrium partition coefficient by means of the formula

$$\overline{C}_{free} = KC_0 \tag{23}$$

where K is the partition coefficient between the tissue and external solution, and C_0 is the concentration of inorganic sulfate in incubating medium or plasma, as the case may be.

In an in vivo experiment, since only a pulse of tracer is injected, the radioactivity due to free ^{35}S in the plasma decays with time, as the tracer first distributes itself throughout the body and then becomes gradually eliminated. If the tissue is very thin (e.g., rabbit articular or disc cartilage) the ^{35}S in the tissue is practically in equilibrium with synovial fluid or plasma throughout the experiment. It is clear, however, that up to time t, N_{free} will no longer be constant, and a mean value has to be obtained.

In larger animals there is another factor to be considered. For an animal such as a large dog, the intervertebral disc is about 5 mm thick, and only at the surface is it in tracer equilibrium with the plasma. Here, the rate of transport of tracer into the tissue also has to be taken into account, and the disc cannot be treated as one well-mixed compartment.

Because the profile of free tracer in the tissue will change with time, as tracer slowly diffuses into the tissue, the counts of incorporated tracer will vary correspondingly throughout the tissue, even if the incorporation rate does not vary with position. Therefore, to obtain Q at any site within the tissue, the variation of free tracer concentration with time at that site needs to be known, as well as the total counts due to incorporated tracer. Figure 15 shows the variation in radioactivity due to free and incorporated tracer in several areas of a dog's disc as a function of time.[7]

2. In Vivo Studies

Using the above procedures, the values given in Table 3 were obtained for the rates of GAG synthesis and turnover rates for rabbit and dog discs as well as, for comparison, for articular cartilage. The turnover rates calculated from the rates of synthesis were verified for rabbits by long-term in vivo studies of the decay of ^{35}S tracer with time up to periods of 1 year.

As can be seen from Table 3, the turnover rates in the disc are very similar to those in cartilage and are very dependent on the age of the animal, varying by more than an order of magnitude from the young to the adult rabbit. The overall rate for GAG synthesis in the adult is slow.   There is unfortunately no information available at the present time on the rates of synthesis in either normal or diseased human discs, where it is obvious that in vitro methods would have to be used.

3. In Vitro Studies

In vitro methods for measuring (^{35}S) sulfate incorporation in articular cartilage have been reviewed by Maroudas and Evans[19] and Maroudas.[44] These techniques cannot be applied directly to the slices of intervertebral discs because these swell significantly and lose PGs during incubation.[45]

Recently, an in vitro method has been developed by Bayliss et al.,[46] consisting of the incubation of disc slices in dialysis tubing surrounded by appropriate ^{35}S-containing medium,

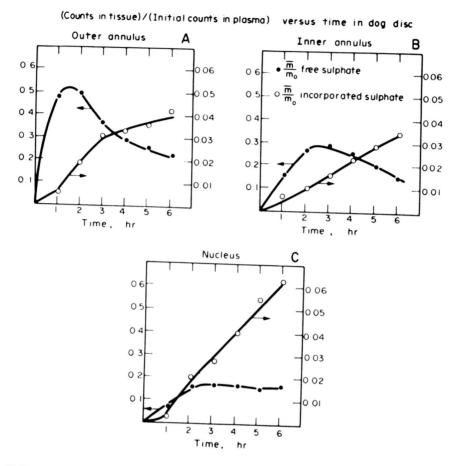

FIGURE 15. Variations of free sulfate and incorporated sulfate tracer concentrations with time in (A) the outer annulus, (B) the inner annulus, and (C) the nucleus. (From Urban, J.P.G. et al., *Biorheology,* 15, 203, 1978. With permission.)

Table 3
RATES OF PROTEOGLYCAN SYNTHESIS AND TURNOVER IN DISCS AND CARTILAGE

Animal	Synthesis rate (mmol/hr/g of tissue $\times 10^6$)	Mean turnover time (days)
Young rabbit (4 weeks)		
Articular cartilage	200	16
Nucleus	140	27
Annulus	175	14
Old rabbit (2 years)		
Articular cartilage	12	340
Nucleus	35	250
Annulus	15	320
Adult dog (greyhound)		
Articular cartilage	12.5	280
Nucleus	15.5	680
Annulus (inner)	18.5	420

with additions of various amounts of polyethylene glycol (PEG) to prevent swelling. By this procedure, Bayliss et al.[46] found for rabbits' discs rates similar to those obtained in vivo and given in Table 3. This method is now being used by Urban[55] for human discs obtained postoperatively, and the preliminary results of synthesis rates are similar to those obtained for human articular cartilage by Maroudas.[44]

An important aspect of the recent in vitro studies on sulfate metabolism in the disc and articular cartilage relates to the observation that the rate of incorporation is highly dependent on applied pressure and hydration.[47,48] Bayliss et al.[46] found that the rate of GAG measured in swollen disc slices was less than half that measured in slices maintained at their in vivo water content. Synthesis rates were also significantly reduced when the hydration of the slice was decreased. Consequently, if measured rates of GAG synthesis are to be related to those found in vivo, the tissue must be maintained at in vivo hydrations. The methods described by Schneiderman et al.[47,48] and Bayliss et al.[46] enable hydration of cartilage and disc slices to be controlled during incubation. Thus, not only can GAG synthesis rates be measured in vitro under in vivo matrix concentrations, but also the effect of hydration and hence of changes in pericellular environment on the production of matrix macromolecules can be systematically studied.

C. Oxygen and Glucose Metabolism

Studies of basal metabolism in cartilaginous tissues have been extremely few in number, possibly because there are a number of inherent procedural difficulties. As far as the large and avascular intervertebral disc is concerned, the subject is clearly of great importance. Accordingly, special methods were developed by the present author and her past collaborators, and this work will now be described in some detail.[43]

1. Oxygen Consumption in the Canine Discs

Oxygen consumption was measured by means of two types of apparatus: (1) an oxygen electrode made into a probe that could be inserted into the nucleus, both in vivo and in vitro;[49] and (2) the Gilson® respirometer[50] for use in vitro on excised tissue specimens. Since the oxygen concentration in the nucleus is very low (see next section) special attention was paid to the variation of oxygen consumption with concentration. The curves of oxygen consumption vs. concentration are shown in Figure 16. The results of oxygen consumption obtained in vitro using the probe are much lower than those obtained in vivo (Figure 16A). However, when they are corrected for the swelling of the tissue, the new values lie close to those measured in vivo throughout the range of oxygen tensions tested (Figure 16A). This good agreement between the oxygen consumption obtained in vivo and in vitro shows that, unlike GAG synthesis,[46] the basic cell metabolism does not appear to be affected by the change in the cellular environment brought about by swelling and loss of PGs in vitro. This is an important finding in relation to possible in vitro studies on the human disc. The results also show that the oxygen consumption is not dependent on oxygen concentration until a very low concentration level is reached (around 4 mmHg).

The Gilson® setup suffers from the disadvantage that the oxygen tension is measured in the solution surrounding the tissue rather than in the tissue itself. As a result of the concentration gradients within the tissue, at low oxygen concentrations, the overall rate of oxygen consumption by the tissue is liable to be underestimated, while the actual local oxygen concentration will be overestimated. It is therefore no surprise that at low oxygen concentration the curve for oxygen consumption lies below that obtained with the oxygen probe (Figure 16B). Since lactic acid production and carbon dioxide evolution have also been studied under similar conditions, it is important to realize that the oxygen tensions measured in the medium do not represent the real concentrations within the tissue.

Although it is the low oxygen concentration range that is of direct physiological interest,

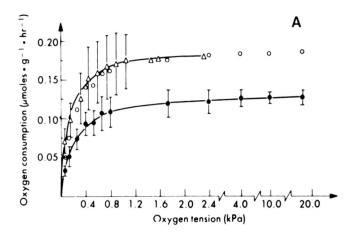

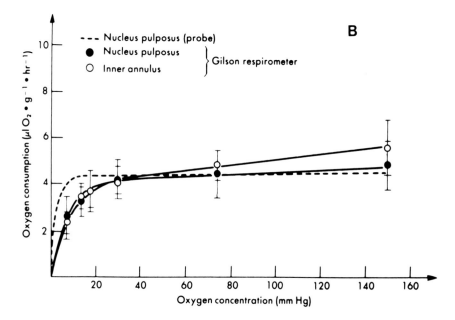

FIGURE 16. (A) Mean O^2 consumption vs. oxygen tension using an oxygen electrode probe. The upper curve represents in vivo determinations; the lower curve represents in vitro results. (○, In vitro results corrected by swelling factor.) (B) Mean oxygen consumption vs. concentration obtained in vitro in a Gilson® respirometer. (- - -, Curve representing results corrected for tissue swelling in vitro.) (From Holm, S. et al., *Connect. Tissue Res.*, 8, 101, 1981. With permission.)

the values at the higher tensions, which are likely to be more accurate, can be used for the purpose of comparison with the oxygen consumptions of other tissues. It should be noted that most published data have in fact been obtained at oxygen tensions of 20.9%, and therefore the comparison will be appropriate. Inspection of Table 3 shows that the oxygen consumption values for the canine disc are comparable, when expressed on a per cell basis, with those for other avascular tissues. On the other hand, the highly vascularized tissues, such as liver and kidney, have consumption rates more than one order of magnitude higher.

Although oxygen consumption is very low in the disc, nevertheless, since the latter is an avascular tissue, diffusion across it results in the formation of considerable concentration gradients, with some regions that are relatively far from the supply route (for example, the center of the nucleus or the inner annulus) having a very low oxygen concentration indeed.

Table 4

**RATES OF GLYCOLYSIS IN THE NUCLEUS PULPOSUS OBTAINED AFTER
INCUBATIONS AT VARIOUS OXYGEN TENSION LEVELS, INCLUDING
VALUES OF THE OXYGEN CONSUMPTION RATES OBTAINED IN THE
GILSON® RESPIROMETER**

Oxygen tension (kPa)	Oxygen consumption rate (Q; μmol/g wet tissue/hr)	Glucose consumption (μmol/g wet tissue/hr)	Lactic acid production (μmol/g wet tissue/hr)	Carbon dioxide production (μmol/g wet tissue/hr)
0.3	0.039	3.3	6.4	0.042
0.9	0.10	3.3	6.4	0.075
1.8	0.13	2.9	6.0	0.13
3.9	0.165	2.7	5.1	0.17
9.8	0.18	2.3	4.5	0.17
19.9	0.19	2.3	4.6	0.17

2. Lactic Acid and Carbon Dioxide Production in the Canine Discs

The results obtained by Holm et al.[43] are shown in Table 4. The oxygen consumption data that were obtained in the Gilson® respirometer are given in the same table and are seen to tally with those of carbon dioxide production. Even at the highest oxygen tension, the proportion of glucose that was converted to carbon dioxide was only 1.5% of the glucose converted to lactic acid. However, although only so small a fraction of glucose was undergoing oxidation to carbon dioxide, the energy provided by this process must constitute about 40% of the total energy produced. The reason for this is that, per mole of glucose, complete oxidation gives rise to 36 mol of ATP, while anaerobic glycolysis produces only 2 mol of ATP.

Since there is approximately a 40% increase in the rate of lactic acid production as the oxygen tension decreases from 9.3 to 0.9 kPa (70 to 7 mmHg), it appears that the cells within the nucleus are able to adjust their rate of glycolysis in such a way as to maintain a constant energy production, whatever the prevailing oxygen tension. With regard to the in vivo situation, this would imply that in the central region of the nucleus, where the oxygen concentration is usually below 1.3 kPa (10 mmHg; see the next section), the glucose consumption and the production of lactic acid are some 25% to 30% higher than near the endplate, where the tension is in the range of 5.3 to 6.7 kPa (40 to 50 mmHg). The rate of production of lactic acid in the canine nucleus pulposus appears to be higher than in the canine articular cartilage for which values around 2 μmol/g/hr were obtained under high oxygen tensions. On a per cell basis the difference is much greater, since the disc has a much lower cell density than articular cartilage (14,000 and 39,000 cells per cubic millimeter, respectively).[42] The mean value obtained by Bywaters[51] for adult human cartilage was 1.5 μmol lactic acid per gram of cartilage (cell density given as 44,000 cells per cubic millimeter) and for rabbit cartilage 6.4 μmol per gram of cartilage (cell density, 128,000 cells per cubic millimeter). For rat epiphyseal cartilage the value of lactic acid production is 6.0 μmol/g of cartilage per hour, and for rabbit corneal stroma a figure of 2.0 μmol/g/hr has been given. It thus appears that the nucleus pulposus produces more lactic acid per cell than a number of other similar connective tissues.

D. Oxygen and Lactate Concentration Profiles

1. Measurement in the Canine Discs

Following measurements of oxygen consumption and lactic acid production in the canine discs, Holm et al.[43] made a study of oxygen and lactic acid concentrations. Oxygen concentrations were measured in vivo using an oxygen electrode at various positions in the disc,

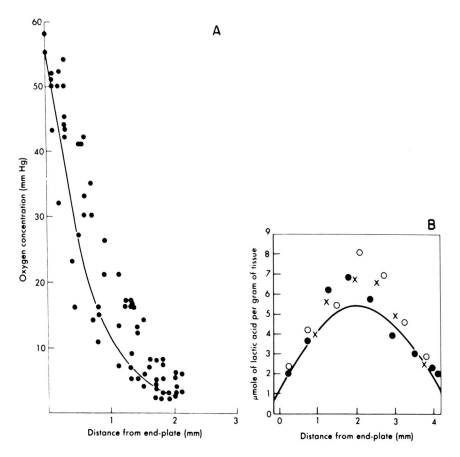

FIGURE 17.   (A) Oxygen concentration profile across the canine nucleus. (●, Experimental points;
—, predicted curve). (B) Lactic acid concentration profile across the nucleus, (○, L4; ×, ●,
L5; —, calculated profile.) (From Holm, S. et al., *Connect. Tissue Res.*, 8, 101, 1981. With permission.)

within both the nucleus pulposus and the annulus fibrosus. Lactic acid concentrations were
determined in slices cut from the nucleus pulposus exicsed from spines frozen immediately
after the dogs had been killed.

The oxygen concentrations were found to vary considerably with position within the
intervertebral disc, being highest near the periphery of the annulus and the end-plate and
lowest in the center of the nucleus and inner annulus. Thus, in the nucleus the oxygen
tension was about 8.0 kPa (60 mmHg) close to the end-plate, decreasing to 0.3 to 1.1 kPa
(2 to 8 mmHg) in the center (Figure 17A). There was very little decrease in oxygen concentrations with increasing distance from the end-plate in the outer part of the annulus, thus
confirming the findings that in this region the end-plate is almost totally impermeable.

Within the nucleus the lactate concentrations were around 1.5 to 2.5 mol/g of wet tissue
near the end-plate, while in the central part they were 5 to 8 μmol/g. There is thus a steep
rise in lactate concentration with the distance from regions in contact with blood vessels
(Figure 17B).

The high lactate levels that are observed, particularly in the center of the larger discs,
must be associated with a lowering of pH. Thus, a lactate concentration of 10 μmol/g of
tissue would lead to pH values about 1 unit lower than in plasma, where the lactate concentration is about 1 μmol/mℓ.

2. Theoretical Calculations

It has been shown that transport by diffusion into the nucleus of the intervertebral disc from the blood vessels beneath the cartilaginous end-plate can be approximated by a one-dimensional diffusion equation. For a steady state diffusion of a metabolite under a concentration gradient set up by the metabolizing cells, the relevant equation is

$$\overline{D} \cdot \frac{d^2C}{dx^2} - R = 0 \qquad (24)$$

where D is the diffusion coefficient in the disc, C is the concentration, x is the distance from the center of the nucleus, and R is the rate of consumption (or production) of the given metabolite.

Using the above equation and the measured values of R as well as of the appropriate partition and diffusion coefficients, it was possible to calculate the expected concentration profiles of both oxygen and lactic acid across the dog's nucleus pulposus and compare them with the experimental results (Figure 17).

There was good agreement between the theoretically calculated oxygen and lactate profiles in the nucleus and the experimental points, although in the central nucleus lactate levels were slightly higher than predicted, probably because the dependence of lactic acid production on oxygen concentration had not been taken into consideration. This agreement confirmed once again that diffusion is the major mechanism whereby nutrients are supplied to the intervertebral disc. If fluid flow resulting from the pumping during walking were a significant contributor to solute transport, one would have anticipated much smaller concentration gradients to be present than those predicted from pure diffusion theory. It should be noted in this connection that, although during the oxygen tension measurements the dogs were under anesthesia and were therefore immobile, the lactate profiles were obtained on dogs that had been left free to move about right up to the time of death. Since the spines were excised and frozen immediately after death, the lactate profiles that were observed must represent fairly closely in the in vivo conditions. The fact that the lactate profiles are certainly as steep as the theoretical profiles thus constitutes strong evidence that the diffusional mechanism, and not fluid flow, is the controlling factor in solute transport in the disc.

3. Extrapolation to the Human Disc

The agreement between the theoretically calculated oxygen and lactate concentration profiles and the experimental results in the canine disc give us the possibility of predicting the profiles in the human disc and, for comparison, in human articular cartilage.

Figure 18 shows such profiles, calculated on the basis of two major assumptions: (1) that the metabolic rates can be extrapolated from the canine to the human articular cartilage and from the canine to the human nucleus pulposus by taking into account the relative cell densities, and (2) that the permeability of the bone-nucleus interface is the same in the two species.

It is clear that if these two assumptions are correct, the lactate concentration in the human nucleus is still higher than in the dog and the concentration of oxygen still lower. Thus, in a region containing 60% of the nucleus (a region at a distance of 2 mm or more from the end-plates) the lactate concentration is higher than 8 mmol/g as compared with 1 to 2 mmol/g near the end-plates. The oxygen concentration drops very steeply with distance from the end-plates. At 1 mm from the latter it has dropped to 10% of its interfacial value. In articular cartilage, while the concentration profiles are also present, they are not nearly as dramatic as in the disc, particularly if one takes into consideration the fractional distances involved in the two cases.

The high lactic acid concentration in the central region of the disc will lead to a decrease in pH, as discussed in Section VI.D.1.

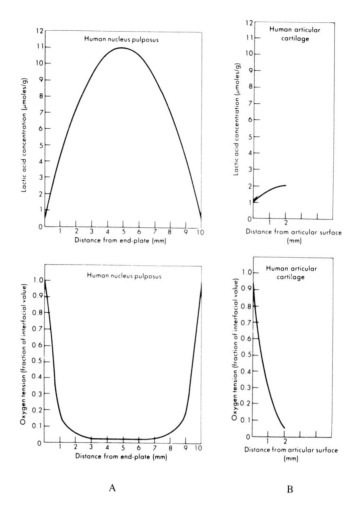

FIGURE 18. Estimated oxygen and lactic acid concentration profiles in human nucleus pulposus (A) and human articular cartilage (B). (From Maroudas, A., Nutrition and metabolism of the intervertebral disc, in *Proceedings of the Workshop of Idiopathic Low Back Pain*, White, A. A., Ed., P. Mosley, Fresno, Calif., 1982. With permission.)

E. Effects of Long-Term Changes in Mechanical Stress on Nutrition and Metabolism

While water flow as such does not significantly influence the transport of essential nutrients, there is recent evidence in the literature, as summarized by Urban and Holm,[52] that long-term alterations in mechanical stress have an effect on the disc's metabolism. Thus, Holm and Nachemson[53] reported that in the discs of the fused section of dog spines, where mechanical stress and movements were reduced, there was a decrease in metabolic activity, whereas in the discs of dogs which had been vigorously exercised for long periods of time (3 months), there was both an increase in the metabolic activity and in the supply of small solutes (charged and uncharged).[54] Urban and Holm[52] suggested that these changes could result from changes in the contact area between disc and blood supply — exercise increasing this contact and thus improving nutrition, while fusion results in a diminution of these blood contacts. The reduced supply of nutrients in fused discs would lead to cellular inactivity or death. On the other hand, the cells could also be reacting to the changed environment, both mechanical and chemical, resulting from mechanical stress. Further work is necessary to confirm these effects and distinguish between the possible causes.

VII. SUMMARY

The knowledge that has been derived from in vitro and in vivo studies of the metabolism and nutrition of the intervertebral disc over the past decade can be summarized as follows.

Metabolites are transported into the disc via two routes: (1) from the blood vessels surrounding the periphery of the annulus and (2) from the blood supply beneath the hyaline cartilage at the bone-disc interface. The permeability of the vertebral end-plate is highest in the region of the nucleus and lowest in the outer annulus. In the canine disc, about 40% of the total end-plate area is estimated to be permeable, although in the region of the nucleus the permeable fraction is as much as 80%. Unfortunately, until now, no quantitative studies have been made of the permeability of the bone-disc interface in human discs, although qualitative work has shown a pattern similar to that observed in the dog.

Diffusion has been found to be the main transport mechanism for small solutes into the intervertebral disc. The important parameters are the partition coefficient, describing the equilibrium distribution of solutes between plasma and disc matrix and the diffusion coefficients, defining the mobility of the solutes. It was found that the diffusion and partition coefficients measured in vitro can be used to describe quantitatively the in vivo transport.

The partition coefficients depend on the size and charge of the solute. Small uncharged solutes have partition coefficients close to unity, i.e., their equilibrium concentration in the disc water is similar to that in the plasma phase in contact. Since the disc matrix has a net negative charge, negatively charged solutes are excluded to a certain extent and have a lower concentration in the disc than in the surrounding plasma. The opposite is true for cations. Their concentration in the disc is always greater than in plasma. The magnitude of the above effects depends on the concentration of the negatively charged fixed groups, and hence on the PG concentration in the tissue. The charge effects are therefore more pronounced in young than in aged discs and vary considerably with location within the disc. Although little work has been done on the penetration of large solutes into the disc, the indications are that they are practically excluded from the nucleus and inner annulus due to the steric effects of PGs whose concentration is high in these regions.

As far as the mobility of the solutes in the disc is concerned, they move more slowly through the disc matrix than in free solution. This is due to the presence of solids within the tissue (collagen and PG) which act as obstacles and lead to an increased tortuosity. The solute has to move through a longer path to cover the distance it would traverse in free solution. The diffusion coefficients of small solutes in the disc — whether the solutes are charged or not — thus have values equal to about 40 to 60% of their values in water. Tortuosity increases with the concentration of solids in the matrix. Thus, solute diffusion coefficients in the annulus are lower than in the more highly hydrated nucleus. There is also a decrease in the diffusion coefficients with age. However, the effect of hydration on the diffusivities is not very large. Moreover, the decrease during aging is offset by a decreased thickness of the discs.

Because the partition coefficients of solutes depend on the local fixed charge density, the relative importance of the two supply routes into the disc will be different for different solutes. Thus, for small, uncharged solutes the two routes into the disc will be of equal importance. For cations, the route via the end-plate is the more effective, but the amount of anions supplied through the periphery of the annulus will be higher than that transported through the end-plate. It should be noted that the relative rates of transport of cations and anions into the disc through the two routes will thus also depend on the relative PG concentrations in the different regions of the disc.

The direct effect of fluid flow accompanying changes in posture and applied load on the transport of small solutes is negligible, since the hydraulic permeability of the disc matrix is very low, while the solute diffusivities are high. However, in the case of the larger solutes whose diffusivities are low, the effect of fluid flow is probably of some significance.

The rates of synthesis of PGs in the discs of adult dogs are of the same order of magnitude as in articular cartilage, and there are strong indications that this is also the case for human discs. Hence the turnover time of the PG in the latter should be of the order of 2 to 3 years. In young animals, the turnover is much more rapid. Recent work has shown the rate of PG synthesis to be very sensitive to the local conditions prevailing in the extracellular matrix, particularly the hydration.

The basal cell metabolism in the disc is mainly anaerobic. Oxygen respiration rates obtained in the nucleus and inner annulus are low but of the same order of magnitude on a per cell basis as those obtained for articular cartilage and those reported for other cartilaginous tissues. Lactic acid production, on the other hand, appears to be higher. The oxygen consumption rates were found to be tension dependent at low oxygen concentrations.

The oxygen concentration in the central part of the dog's disc is very low, in the region of 0.2 to 1.0 kPa (2 to 8 mmHg), and the lactate concentration is high, about 6 to 8 mmol/g.

The knowledge that diffusion is the main mechanism of solute transport in the disc gives us the possibility of calculating the concentrations of different metabolites in the human disc provided their rates of production or utilization have been determined. Thus, assuming that the metabolic rates can be extrapolated from the canine to the human disc by taking into account the relative cell densities, we have estimated that in the central nucleus the oxygen concentrations would be around 0.5 to 1.3 kPa (4 to 10 mmHg), and the lactate concentrations would be in the range of 10 to 15 mmol/g of tissue, that is, 10 to 5 times higher than in plasma. The resulting lowering of pH of 1 unit or more might, in turn, adversely affect cell metabolism in the central nucleus and might also enhance the activity of pH-dependent degradative enzymes, such as cathepsin D or B.

Apart from the specific effects of low pH, it should be noted that in a general sense the cells in the central part of a large disc are in an especially precarious situation for the following reason. Since in that region a low oxygen tension prevails, an increased rate of glycolysis appears to be needed to satisfy the energy requirements of the cells. This, in turn, implies a greater demand for glucose. However, in a large disc, the extra glucose may not be forthcoming, and the cells may therefore be unable to satisfy fully their energy requirements.

An important parameter in any disc in relation to its nutritional status is the permeability of the bone-end-plate interface, that is, the area of contact between the blood vessels and the end-plate. Unfortunately, the validity of the in vitro methods for quantifying the latter has not been confirmed up to the present. Since the permeability of the end-plate has been quantified in the dog in vivo, in vitro methods should now be developed and tested in this animal before they are applied to the human disc. Thereafter a post-mortem survey of human discs should be made involving the measurement of the disc dimensions, the permeable fraction of the bone-disc interface, and the cellularity of the different regions of the disc. The nutritional requirements could then be compared with the calculated solute availability at different points in the disc, and possibly a correlation with the degree of disc degeneration could be obtained.

REFERENCES

1. **Urban. J. P. G.,** Fluid and Solute Transport in the Intervertebral Disc, Ph.D. thesis, London University, London, England, 1977.
2. **Urban, J. P. G. and Maroudas, A.,** The chemistry of the intervertebral disc in relation to its physiological function and requirements, *Clin. Rheum. Dis.,* 6, 51, 1980.

3. **Urban, J. P. G. and Maroudas, A.,** Measurement of swelling pressures and fluid flow in the intervertebral disc with reference to creep, in *Engineering Aspects of the Spine,* Institution of Mechanical Engineers Publications, London, 1981.

4. **Maroudas, A.,** Swelling pressures in cartilaginous tissues, in *Studies in Joint Disease,* Vol. 1, Maroudas, A. and Holborow, J., Eds., Pitman Medical, London, 1980, chap. 3.

5. **Maroudas, A. and Venn, M.,** Swelling of normal and osteoarthrotic femoral head cartilage, *Ann. Rheum. Dis.,* 36, 399, 1977.

6. **Maroudas, A.,** Physical chemistry of cartilage and the intervertebral disc, in *The Joints and Synovial Fluid,* Sokoloff, L., Ed., Academic Press, New York, 1980, 239.

7. **Urban, J. P. G., Holm, S., and Maroudas, A.,** Diffusion of small solutes into the intervertebral disc, *Biorheology,* 15, 203, 1978.

8. **Maroudas, A.,** Physico-chemical properties of articular cartilage, in *Adult Articular Cartilage,* 2nd ed., Freeman, M. A. R., Ed., Pitman Medical, London, 1973, 131.

9. **Maroudas, A. and Bannon, C.,** Measurement of swelling pressure in cartilage and comparison with the osmotic pressure of constituent proteoglycans, *Biorheology,* 18, 619, 1981.

10. **Urban, J. P. G. and McMullin, J. F.,** Swelling pressure of the intervertebral disc: influence of proteoglycan and collagen contents, *Biorheology,* 22, 145, 1985.

11. **Katz, E. P., Wachtel, E. J., and Maroudas, A.,** Extrafibrillar proteoglycans osmotically regulate the molecular packing of collagen in cartilage, *Biochim. Biophys. Acta,* 882, 136, 1986.

12. **Weinberg, P., Maroudas, A., Katz, E. P., Wachtel, E. J., and Schneiderman, R.,** Intrafibrillar water in cartilaginous tissues, *Calcif. Tissue Res.,* in press.

13. **Ziv, I. and Maroudas, A.,** Variation in some physical chemical properties in the human intervertebral disc with age, in preparation.

14. **Urban. J. and Maroudas, A.,** The measurement of fixed charge density in the intervertebral disc, *Biochim. Biophys. Acta,* 568, 166, 1979.

15. **Maroudas, A. and Thomas, H.,** A simple physicochemical micromethod for determining fixed anionic groups in connective tissue, *Biochim. Biophys. Acta,* 215, 214, 1970.

16. **Venn, M. and Maroudas, A.,** Chemical composition of normal and osteoarthrotic femoral head cartilage, *Ann. Rheum. Dis.,* 36, 121, 1977.

17. **Urban, J. P. G. and Maroudas, A.,** Swelling of the intervertebral disc in vitro, *Connect. Tissue Res.,* 9, 1, 1981.

18. **Hellfrich, F.,** *Ion Exchange,* McGraw-Hill, New York, 1962, chap. 5 and 6.

19. **Maroudas, A. and Evans, H.,** In vitro study of sulphate diffusion and incorporation by adult human articular cartilage, *Biochim. Biophys, Acta,* 338, 265, 1974.

20. **Ogston, A. G.,** The biological functions of the glycosaminoglycans, in *Chemistry and Molecular Biology of the Intercellular Matrix,* Vol. 3, Balazs, E. A., Ed., Academic Press, London, 1970, 1231.

21. **Pikal, M. J. and Bloyd, G. E.,** Tracer diffusion of HTO and simple ions in aqueous solutions of sodium *p*-ethylbenzenesulphate, *J. Phys. Chem.,* 77, 2918, 1973.

22. **Maroudas, A.,** Transport of large solutes through cartilage, *J. Anat.,* 120, 335, 1976.

23. **Crank, J. and Park, G. S.,** Methods of measurement, in *Diffusion in Polymers,* Crank, J. and Park, G. S., Eds., Academic Press, London, 1968, 16.

24. **Maroudas, A., Weinberg, P. D., Parker, K. H., and Winlove, C. P.,** The distributions and diffusivities of small ions in chondroitin sulphate, hyaluronate, and proteoglycan, *Biophys. Chem.,* in press.

25. **Mackie, J. S. and Meares, P.,** Diffusion of electrolytes in cation exchange resin, *Proc. R. Soc. London Ser. A,* 232, 498, 1955.

26. **Paulson, S. and Sylven, B.,** Biophysical and physiological investigations on cartilage and other mesemchymal tissues. III. The diffusion rate of various substances in normal bovine nucleus pulposus, *Biochim. Biophys. Acta,* 7, 217, 1951.

27. **Nachemson, A., Lewin, T., Maroudas, A., and Freeman, M. A. R.,** In vitro diffusion of dye through the endplates and the annulus fibrosus of human lumbar intervertebral discs, *Acta Orthop. Scand.,* 41, 589, 1970.

28. **Holm, S., Maroudas, A., Urban, J. P. G., and Nachemson, A.,** Nutrition of the intervertebral disc: an in vivo study of solute transport, *Clin. Orthop. Relat. Res.,* 178, 1977.

29. **Faxen, H.,** Der Widerstand gegen die Bewegung einer stamen Kugel in einer Zatten Flussigkeit die zwischen zwei parallenebenen Wanden eingeschlossen ist, *Ann. Phys. (Leipzig),* 4, 68, 1922.

30. **Ogston, A. G., Preston, B. N., and Wells, S. O.,** On the transport of compact particles through solutions of chain polymers, *Proc. R. Soc. London Ser. A,* 333, 297, 1973.

31. **Brodin, H.,** Paths of nutrition in articular cartilage and intervertebral discs, *Acta Orthop. Scand.,* 24, 177, 1955.

32. **Lewin, T., Nachemson, A., Maroudas, A., and Freeman, M. A. R.,** In vitro diffusion of dye through the end-plates and the annulus fibrosis of human lumbar intervertebral discs, *Acta Orthop. Scand.,* 41, 589, 1970.

33. **Urban, J. and Maroudas, A.,** Measurement of swelling pressure and fluid flow in the intervertebral disc with reference to creep, in *Engineering Aspects of the Spine,* Institution of Mechanical Engineers Publications, London, 1980.
34. **Maroudas, A.,** Mechanisms of fluid transport in cartilaginous tissues, in *Tissue Nutrition and Viability,* Hargens, A. R., Ed., Springer-Verlag, New York, 1986, chap. 3.
35. **Nachemson, A. and Elfstrom, G.,** Intravital dynamic pressure measurements in lumbar discs, *Scand. J. Rehab. Med.,* Suppl. 2, 1970.
36. **Andersson, G. B. J.,** Measurement of loads on the lumbar spine, in *Idiopathic Low Back Pain,* White, A. A. and Gordon, S. L., Eds., C. V. Mosby, St. Louis, 1982, 220.
37. **Adams, M. A. and Hutton, W. C.,** The mechanics of the prolapsed intervertebral disc, a hyperflexion injury, *Spine,* 7, 184, 1982.
38. **Hickey, D. S. and Hukins, D. W. L.,** The relationship between the structure of the annulus fibrosus and the function and failure of the intervertebral disc, *Spine,* 5, 106, 1980.
39. **Urban, J. P. G., Maroudas, A., Bayliss, M. T., and Dillon, J.,** Swelling pressures of proteoglycans at the concentrations found in cartilaginous tissues, *Biorheology,* 16, 447, 1979.
40. **Fatt, I. and Goldstick, T. K.,** The dynamics of water transport in swelling membranes, *J. Colloid Sci.,* 20, 962, 1965.
41. **Urban, J. P. G., Holm, S., Maroudas, A., and Nachemson, A.,** Nutrition of the intervertebral disc: effect of fluid flow in solute transport, *Clin. Orthop. Relat. Res.,* 170, 209, 1982.
42. **Maroudas, A., Nachemson, A., Stockwell, R. A., and Urban, J. P. G.,** Factors involved in the nutrition of human lumbar intervertebral disc: cellularity and diffusion of glucose in vitro, *J. Anat.,* 120, 113, 1975.
43. **Holm, S., Maroudas, A., Urban, J. P. G., Selstam, G., and Nachemson, A.,** Nutrition of the intervertebral disc, solute transport and metabolism, *Connect. Tissue Res.,* 8, 101, 1981.
44. **Maroudas, A.,** Metabolism and turnover of cartilaginous tissues, in *Studies in Joint Disease,* Vol. 1., Maroudas, A. and Holborow, J., Eds., Pitman Medical, London, 1980, 59.
45. **Urban, J. P. G. and Maroudas, A.,** Swelling of intervertebral disc in vitro, *Connect. Tissue Res.,* 9, 1, 1981.
46. **Bayliss, M. Y., Urban, J. P. G., Johnstone, B., and Holm, S.,** An in vitro method for measuring synthesis rates in the intervertebral disc, *J. Orthop. Res.,* in press.
47. **Schneiderman, R., Keret, D., and Maroudas, A.,** Effects of mechanically and osmotically applied compression on sulphate incorporation in human articular cartilage, in *Degenerative Joints,* Vol. 2, Verbruggen, G. and Veys, E. M., Eds., Elsevier, Amsterdan, 1985, 21.
48. **Schneiderman, R., Keret, D., and Maroudas, A.,** The effects of mechanical and osmotic pressure on the rate of glycosaminoglycan synthesis in the human adult femoral head cartilage: an in vitro study, *J. Orthop. Res.,* in press.
49. **Ejesmar, A. and Holm, S.,** Oxygen tension measurements in the intervertebral disc, a methodological and experimental study, *Upsalla J. Med. Sci.,* 84, 83, 1979.
50. **Gilson, W. E.,** Differential respirometer of simplified and improved design, *Science,* 141, 531, 1963.
51. **Bywaters, E. G. L.,** The metabolism of joint tissues, *J. Pathol. Bacteriol.,* 44, 247, 1937.
52. **Urban, J. P. G. and Holm, S. H.,** Intervertebral disc nutrition as related to spinal movements and fusion, in *Tissue Nutrition and Viability,* Hargens, A. R., Ed., Springer-Verlag, New York, 1986, chap. 5.
53. **Holm, S. and Nachemson, A.,** Nutritional changes in the canine intervertebral disc after spinal fusion, *Clin. Orthop. Relat. Res.,* 169, 243, 1982.
54. **Holm, S. and Nachemson, A.,** Variations in the nutrition of the canine intervertebral disc induced by motion, *Spine,* 8, 866, 1983.
55. **Urban, J. P. G.,** personal communication.

Chapter 10

MECHANICS OF THE INTERVERTEBRAL DISC

Michael A. Adams and William C. Hutton

TABLE OF CONTENTS

I. INTRODUCTION

This chapter describes the forces that act on the intervertebral discs and how the discs respond to them. It begins with a brief account of spinal mechanics (Section II) in order to outline the precise function of the discs. Section III describes the physical and mechanical properties of disc tissues. These are then used to explain the response of the discs to compression, bending, and torsion, in Sections IV, V, and VI, respectively. None of these simple loading patterns causes discs to prolapse, and Section VII shows that complex loading in compression and bending is necessary for prolapse to occur. Mechanical loading causes fluid movements within the discs, and these give rise to time-dependent mechanical properties, as described in Section VIII. Section IX shows how mechanical properties vary with age and spinal level. Finally, Section X suggests how mechanical factors may affect the transportation of metabolites in the disc. Research into disc mechanics has been stimulated by the need to understand and explain low back pain, and consequently most of the experimental data concern lumbar discs. Usually, these data can be applied to thoracic and cervical discs as well. Where such generalizations are considered unwarranted, it is emphasized in the text that the data concern lumbar discs.

II. ROLE OF THE DISC IN THE MECHANICS OF THE SPINE

To a certain extent, the mechanical function of the intervertebral discs can be inferred from the anatomy of the spine. Obviously, the discs must transmit compressive forces from one vertebra to the next, while at the same time allowing a limited amount of movement between vertebrae. However, anatomical inferences can be misleading (see Section II.D below), and it is necessary to use the results of mechanical experiments on cadaveric spines in order to describe the precise role of the discs in spinal mechanics.

A. Compression of the Spine

The intervertebral compressive force is defined here as that force which acts down the long axis of the spine, at right angles to the intervertebral discs. The force is due to superincumbent body weight (which can be effectively increased when the body is acclerated or decelerated), and to tensile forces in the muscles and ligaments surrounding the spine. These latter forces are difficult to estimate, and they cannot be neglected even in relaxed postures since a certain amount of antagonistic muscle activity is required to stabilize the erect spine.[1] However, there is a method of directly measuring the compressive force on the lumbar spine of living people.[2,3] A needle bearing a miniature pressure transducer is inserted into the nucleus pulposus of a lumbar disc (usually L3—4) of an active volunteer. The pressure readings obtained need to be calibrated against readings obtained from cadaveric

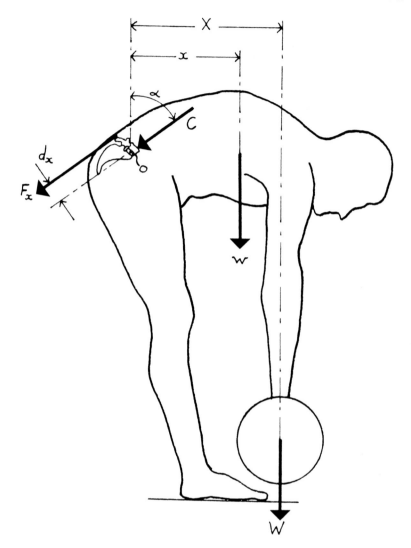

FIGURE 1. Forces acting to compress the lumbar spine. Taking moments about the center of rotation 0, the extensor moment generated by the back muscles ($F_x d_x$) is balanced by the forward bending moment due to the weight lifted (WX) and due to superincumbent body weight (wx). The compressive force on the lumbar spine is $C = F_x + (w + W)$ cosα. (From Hutton, W. C. and Adams, M. A., *Spine*, 7(6), 587, 1982. With permission.)

spinal segments subjected to known compressive forces.[4] Typical values of compressive force obtained by this method and published in 1981 are 250 N when lying supine, 500 N when standing at ease, 700 N when sitting upright, and 1900 N when lifting 10 kg with the back bent.[2] (Earlier published values were too high because of a zero error.)

Evidently, the forces on the lumbar spine increase greatly in forward bending activities. Unfortunately, the experimental technique described above is unsuitable for use in fully flexed postures since the pressure transducer actually measures the hydrostatic pressure in the nucleus pulposus, and this is affected by flexion and extension of the spine.[5] It is necessary to use a simple mathematical model in order to estimate the forces acting in full flexion and heavy lifting (see Figure 1). The calculation shows that when a heavy weight is lifted or carried in the fully flexed position there are high tensile forces in the back muscles which raise the compressive force on the spine to values of 6000 to 9000 N.[6]

The body has a mechanism for lowering these high compressive forces on the spine. By holding the breath and contracting the trunk muscles, it is possible to raise the hydraulic pressure in the abdominal cavity; this then acts like an inflated support to transmit force directly from the upper body to the pelvis, bypassing the spine.[7,8] This effect is difficult to quantify, but calculations suggest that the compressive force on the lumbar spine may be reduced by up to 3000 N[9] or even more.[10]

Most of the compressive force on the spine is resisted by the intervertebral discs since the force acts more or less parallel to the articular surfaces (facets) of the apophyseal joints. However, the facets can resist compression under certain circumstances: it all depends on the height of the disc, and the degree of flexion or extension of the lumbar spine. When a motion segment is wedged and compressed in 2° of extension (in order to simulate some lordotic posture such as erect standing) and is creep loaded to reduce the fluid content of the disc (see Section VIII.B) then the facets resist on average about one sixth of the compressive force.[11] This proportion increases at higher angles of extension or if the disc height is reduced by discectomy.[12] If the disc is grossly degenerated and narrowed, 70% of the compressive force can be resisted by the facets.[11] Occasionally, a small proportion of the compressive force can be resisted by the spinous processes, a phenomenon known as kissing spines.[11] Conversely, flexed postures throw all the compression onto the discs. Only 2° of flexion per lumbar level is needed for this to happen.[11]

B. Shear on the Spine

The intervertebral shear force acts in the midplane of the disc and tends to cause each vertebra to move forward relative to the one below. It cannot be measured directly, but calculations suggest that it can be as great as 750 N in the lumbar spine during forward bending and lifting movements.[13]

In the lumbar spine, the facets are well oriented to resist this shear force. When a motion segment is loaded in combined compression and shear, the facets initially resist about one half to two thirds of the shear force while the disc resists the remainder.[13,14] However, an isolated disc creeps forward in response to sustained loading.[15] In an intact motion segment, the disc's readiness to creep manifests as stress relaxation and causes an increasing proportion of the shear force to be resisted by the facets. It is likely that, in most circumstances in life, most or all of the intervertebral shear force is resisted by the apophyseal joints. The tendency for the neural arch to be bent backward by this force is probably countered by the action of back muscles pulling down on the spinous process.[13]

C. Bending of the Spine

The spine can bend forward (flexion), sideways (lateral flexion), and backward (extension). Typical ranges of motion for healthy adults are shown in Table 1. The range of motion decreases with age[16,17] and is often much reduced in people with back pain.[18] During bending movements, the nucleus pulposus acts rather like a ball bearing, allowing the upper vertebral body to pivot about the lower one, with the annulus fibrosus and intervertebral ligaments resisting the motion. This is an oversimplification, however, since in living people, bending movements involve changes in the shear and compressive forces acting on the spine, so the resulting vertebral movement is a combination of rotation and translation, and the center of rotation moves within the disc during the movement.[45] The three bending movements will now be considered separately.

1. Flexion

Flexion is resisted by compression of the anterior annulus and stretching of the posterior annulus and the ligaments of the neural arch. The position of the center of rotation means that the articular surfaces of the apophyseal joints just glide past each other with no measurable

Table 1
TYPICAL RANGE OF MOTION AT EACH SPINAL LEVEL

Spinal level	Range of motion (degrees)			
	Flexion[a]	Extension[a]	Lateral bending[b]	Axial rotation[b]
C2—3	8		10	9
C3—4	13		11	11
C4—5	12		11	12
C5—6	17		8	10
C6—7	16		7	9
C7—T1	9		4	8
T1—2 to T9—10	4—6		6	4—9
T10—11 to T12—L1	9—12		7—9	2
L1—2	8	5	10	2
L2—3	10	3	11	2
L3—4	12	1	10	3
L4—5	13	2	6	3
L5—S1	9	5	3	2

Note: Values for the cervical and thoracic spine are estimates by White and Panjabi,[84] and values for the lumbar spine are from biplanar X-ray measurements by Pearcy and colleagues.[26,85]

[a] Angles for lumbar spine measured relative to erect standing.
[b] Total movement from right to left.

resistance.[19] (It has been claimed that the bony facets resist flexion,[20] but this is probably an artifact caused by flexing cadaveric specimens in an unphysiological manner.) When a motion segment is subjected to complex loading that simulates forward bending movements in life, then in full flexion, the applied bending moment is resisted by the apophyseal joint capsular ligaments (39% on average), the disc (29%), the interspinous and supraspinous ligaments (19%), and the ligamentum flavum (13%).[19] The whole motion segment can resist a bending moment of about 50 Nm before it sustains damage.[19] However, this is only half of the bending moment exerted by the upper body on the lumbar spine in the toe-touching posture, so it is apparent that the flexed osteoligamentous spine receives considerable support from the back muscles and lumbodorsal fascia. This is confirmed by the fact that living people do not, in practice, flex their spines right up to the elastic limit, but stay about 10° short of this limit.[21]

If a lumbar motion segment is flexed beyond its elastic limit, the first structures to be damaged are the supraspinous and interspinous ligaments,[19] followed by the capsular ligaments and then the intervertebral disc.[22] The mechanics of flexion movements are subject to an interesting diurnal variation.[23] In the early morning, the intervertebral discs have a higher fluid content (see Section VIII.A), and this makes the spine more resistant to forward bending. The back muscles do not fully compensate for this by restricting the range of flexion. Instead they allow the bending stresses on the disc (in particular) and ligaments to increase considerably in the early morning.

2. Lateral Flexion

Anatomical considerations suggest that lateral flexion is resisted by the disc, the intertransverse ligaments, and the apophyseal joint capsular ligaments. However, the part played by each structure has not been quantified by experiment. At small angles of bending (about

2° to 3°) there is negligible resistance from the neural arch, and lumbar discs are less stiff than thoracic discs.[24] Cadaveric experiments have shown that lateral flexion movements can couple with axial rotation movements,[25] but this coupling is not consistent in living people and is probably under muscular control.[26] A component of lateral flexion, when combined with flexion and compression, can play a significant part in the mechanism of disc prolapse (see Section VII).

3. Extension

Extension is resisted by the disc, the apophyseal joints, and (in rare cases) by "kissing" spinous processes. The spine resists small extension movements more than flexion or lateral flexion.[27] Stresses between the apophyseal joint surfaces rise rapidly with increasing extension angle,[11,12] and this bony contact probably limits the movement.

D. Axial Rotation of the Spine

Axial rotation (torsion) is a twisting of the spine about its long axis and is typified by actions such as discus throwing. It is commonly, but incorrectly, thought that bending over and swinging round from side to side involves considerable axial rotation. This kind of movement occurs naturally during digging and in many working tasks, but it is essentially a varying combination of forward and lateral bending rather than axial rotation.

The center of axial rotation is poorly defined, but experiments on cadaveric lumbar motion segments have located it in the posterior half of the disc or in the spinal canal.[28,29] It is not posterior to the apophyseal joints, as might be expected from the orientation of the lumbar facet surfaces (see Figure 2).

The range of movement found in life is shown in Table 1. The marked variation in the range of movement at different spinal levels is probably due to the varying orientation of the apophyseal joints, since bony resistance in the compression facet (Figure 2) limits axial rotation, at least in the lumbar spine.[29] When lumbar motion segments are loaded in combined compression and torsion to simulate full axial rotation movements in life, the apophyseal joints are compressed. The discs resist a proportion of the torque, while the ligaments of the neural arch offer very little resistance.[29] The ligamentous resistance probably increases at other spinal levels, where the range of movement is much greater.

E. Summary: The Mechanical Function of the Disc

The experimental work reviewed above shows that the main function of the intervertebral discs is to transmit compressive force from one vertebral body to the next. Except in lordotic postures, all of the compressive force on the spine goes through the discs. The discs also offer considerable resistance to spinal movements but are protected by the apophyseal joint surfaces from excessive shear, torsion, and extension, and by the ligaments of the neural arch from excessive flexion and lateral flexion. This is summarized in Figure 3.

III. MECHANICAL PROPERTIES OF DISC TISSUES

Mechanically, as well as morphologically, the intervertebral disc consists of two parts, the nucleus pulposus and the annulus fibrosus. The nucleus of a nondegenerated disc is a soft proteoglycan-water gel, loosely held together by a fine network of collagen fibers. The annulus is made of the same constituents, but here the gel is much more firmly held between thick concentric "fences" of collagen which are anchored in the vertebral body end-plates above and below and are cross-linked to each other (Figure 4). The collagen network of the annulus restrains the tendency of the proteoglycan-water gel to absorb water from surrounding tissue and swell up. Thus, the collagen fibers are always in tension, and the gel is always in compression. This arrangement is called prestressing, and it gives the disc its compressive

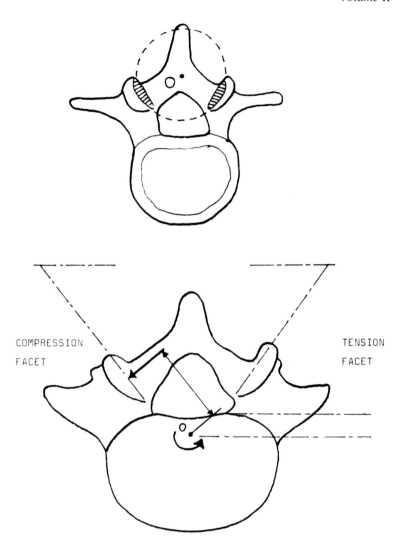

FIGURE 2.   Axial rotation of the lumbar spine. (Top) If it is assumed that the facets do not restrict axial rotation, then the center of rotation 0 will be as shown; however, experiments do not support this. (Bottom) With a center of rotation in the posterior annulus, one apophyseal joint is compressed, and the other is stretched by axial rotation.

stiffness or turgor. The different collagen networks of the annulus and nucleus give these tissues markedly different mechanical properties.

A. Annulus Fibrosus

The tensile properties of annulus fibrosus material have been thoroughly investigated by Galante,[30] and a summary of his results is shown in Table 2. A high value of elongation means the specimen was extensible and not very stiff, while a high value of energy dissipation means the specimen did not show good elastic recovery once the tensile load was removed. Several conclusions can be drawn from this table. First, lines 1 through 3 show that the annulus is much stiffer and stronger and has better elastic recovery when stretched circumferentially compared to when it is stretched vertically (that is, along the long axis of the spine). Evidently, the annulus is able to resist hoop stresses better than a separation of the vertebral end-plates. Second, lines 4 through 7 show that the outer annulus is stiffer and

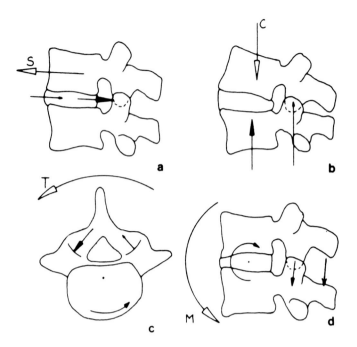

FIGURE 3.   The apophyseal joints and ligaments of the neural arch act in conjunction with the disc to resist (a) shear (S); (b) compression (C); (c) torsion (T); and (d) bending (M). The proportional resistance from each structure is represented by the size of the solid arrowheads. (From Adams, M. A. and Hutton, W. C., *Spine*, 8(3), 328, 1983. With permission.)

has a better elastic recovery than the inner annulus. The anterior annulus is stiffer and has a better elastic recovery than the posterior annulus. In addition, Sonoda[31] has shown that outer annulus material has about twice the tensile strength of inner annulus material. These variations are more difficult to interpret. They may indicate that tensile stresses are normally higher in the outer annulus and anterior annulus. Alternatively, they may reflect the fact that degenerative changes are generally more advanced in the inner and posterior annulus, since degeneration reduces stiffness and elastic recovery (Table 2, lines 10 through 11). Third, lines 8 and 9 show that annulus fibrosus material is viscoelastic and behaves less elastically when deformed slowly (see Section VII).

The compressive properties cannot be tested in the same way since the disrupted collagen network of small samples would allow it to deform and buckle. However, the annulus as a whole is well able to resist high compressive forces directly. This has been demonstrated by compressing cadaveric lumbar discs before and after the removal of the nucleus pulposus and finding little difference in the specimen's stiffness.[32]

B. Nucleus Pulposus

The loose collagen network of the nucleus pulposus allows the material to be easily deformed and separated into pieces, and thus, it is not really suitable for mechanical testing in tension or compression. However, a tensile strength of 0.2 to 0.3 MPa has been reported,[31] and certain other physical characteristics of the material have been described qualitatively.[33] In an adolescent, the nucleus is a viscous semitransparent fluid that flows under its own weight. In the 3rd decade, it is soft and white and shows regions of greater and lesser cohesion that gradually become more exaggerated and coalescent. By about the 5th decade the nucleus usually consists of several discrete fibrous bodies surrounded by softer material

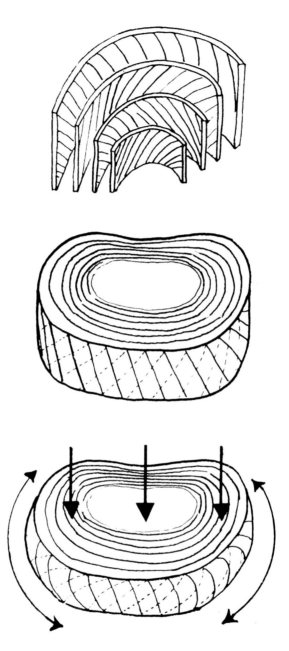

FIGURE 4. Structure of the intervertebral disc. (Top) The concentric lamellae of the annulus are expanded to show the alternating fiber angle. (Center and bottom) Compression of the disc causes height loss, increased radial bulging, and a change in alternating fiber angle. The nucleus pulposus exhibits a hydrostatic pressure and creates a tangential hoop stress in the annulus.

which may contain large fissures or lines of fracture. With old age, and with degeneration, the nucleus becomes dessicated and fibrous.

Table 2
TENSILE PROPERTIES OF THE ANNULUS FIBROSUS[30]

Specimen group	Load (N)	Elongation (mm)	Energy dissipation J/mm³ (× 10⁶)	Tensile strength (MPa)	Elongation at failure (%)
Group 1					
1 with $\theta = 0°$	0.49	0.68	2.45	3.4	25.1
2 with $\theta = \phi$				10.5	31.5
3 with $\theta = 90°$		5.03	23.0	Often < 0.25	
Group 2					
4 Anterior with d = 1 mm	1.96	1.07	10.5		
5 Anterior with d = 4 mm		1.72	18.7		
6 Posterior with d = 1 mm		1.36	10.5		
7 Posterior with d = 4 mm		2.07	19.6		
Group 3					
8 with 0.5-cm/min strain rate	1.96	1.14	12.7		
9 with 5.0-cm/min strain rate		1.16	8.6		
Group 4					
10 Normal discs	1.96	1.03	9.1		
11 Degenerated discs		1.34	15.8		

Note: Specimens were 10 mm long and 2 × 1 mm in cross section. Specimen group 1 shows how the tensile properties vary with orientation. (θ is the angle between the long axis of the specimen and the midplane of the disc; $\theta = \phi$ means that the specimen was cut parallel to the fiber direction.) Specimen group 2 shows the variation with location in the disc. (Anterior, anterior annulus; d, distance from periphery of annulus). Specimen groups 3 and 4 show how the tensile properties vary with strain rate and disc degeneration.

IV. AXIAL LOADING

A. Symmetrical Compression

When the spine is subjected to pure compression, there is an even compressive stress (force per unit area) on the discs,[35] but the annulus and nucleus resist it in different ways. The annulus is relatively rigid and resists compressive stresses directly.[32] It loses height and bulges radially, and this deformation is probably facilitated by a decrease in the angle between the collagen fibers of adjacent lamellae (see Figure 2).[36] Without the support of the nucleus, annular bulging increases considerably.[34,37]

The nucleus, in contrast, behaves like a pressurized fluid. Even when no external forces are applied to a disc, the nucleus exhibits an intrinsic hydrostatic pressure[38] which is caused by the annulus resisting the tendency of the nucleus to absorb tissue fluid and swell up. An external compressive stress raises the pressure in the nucleus and causes the vertebral body end-plates to bulge outward.[39] The nuclear pressure also creates a tangential (hoop) stress in the annulus[4] which decreases with distance from the nucleus (according to the theory of thick-walled pressure cylinders). At high load levels, the outward bulging of the end-plates can account for most of the height lost by the disc.[39] The hydrostatic behavior of the nucleus is demonstrated even in slightly degenerated discs,[40] but is unlikely to persist as degenerative changes become more severe.

It is worth emphasizing that the radial bulging of the annulus is due to direct compression of the annulus and not to the hydrostatic pressure in the nucleus. In fact, when the nuclear pressure is increased by fluid injection, the radial bulge of the annulus decreases.[34] (This is rather like pumping air into a flat tire.)

Like most biological structures, intervertebral discs have nonlinear mechanical properties.[24] This just means that the more they are deformed, the stiffer they become. Nonlinearity can be attributed to the way collagen fibers stretch. At low loads, the fibers are not quite straight, but have bends or kinks in them which gradually straighten out as the load increases. At high loads, the fibers are stretched directly, and the material is then much stiffer. Nonlinearity enables the disc to deform considerably under low loads (and so to act as a shock absorber) without collapsing completely under sudden high loading.

Intervertebral discs are extremely strong in compression, and generally compressive failure of a motion segment occurs in the vertebral bodies, often by a fracture of the end-plate.[41,42] The compressive strength of a lumbar motion segment varies from about 3000 to 11,000 N, depending on the sex, age, and body mass of the cadaver.[9,41,42] Isolated discs have been compressed to failure,[31] and results for cadavers aged between 40 and 59 years are shown in Table 3. At failure, there is a splitting of the posterior annulus, and nucleus pulposus material escapes.

B. Asymmetrical Compression

In life, the lumbar spine is rarely subjected to pure compression as just described. Most standing and sitting postures apply a bending moment as well so that the disc becomes wedged in flexion or extension, as shown in Figure 5. When a disc is compressed while wedged in flexion, the compressive stress is highest on the anterior annulus and lowest on the posterior annulus. Conversely, when a disc is compressed while wedged in extension, the compressive stress is highest on the posterior annulus and lowest on the anterior annulus.[35] These anterior-posterior pressure gradients have not been demonstrated experimentally on young nondegenerated lumbar discs. However, this is probably because such discs are so deformable in the sagittal plane that they need to be flexed or extended to large angles before the gradients become apparent.

Asymmetrical loading causes asymmetrical radial bulging of the disc, with the bulge being more pronounced where the compressive stress is greatest, and reduced or absent on the

Table 3
COMPRESSIVE STRENGTH CHARACTERISTICS OF CADAVERIC INTERVERTEBRAL DISCS[31]

	Cervical discs	Thoracic discs	Lumbar discs
Compressive breaking load (N)	3139	4415—11,282	14,715
Compressive strength (MPa)	10.6	10.3	11.0
Ultimate compression (%)	35	30	35

Note: Discs were from cadavers aged between 40 and 59 years.

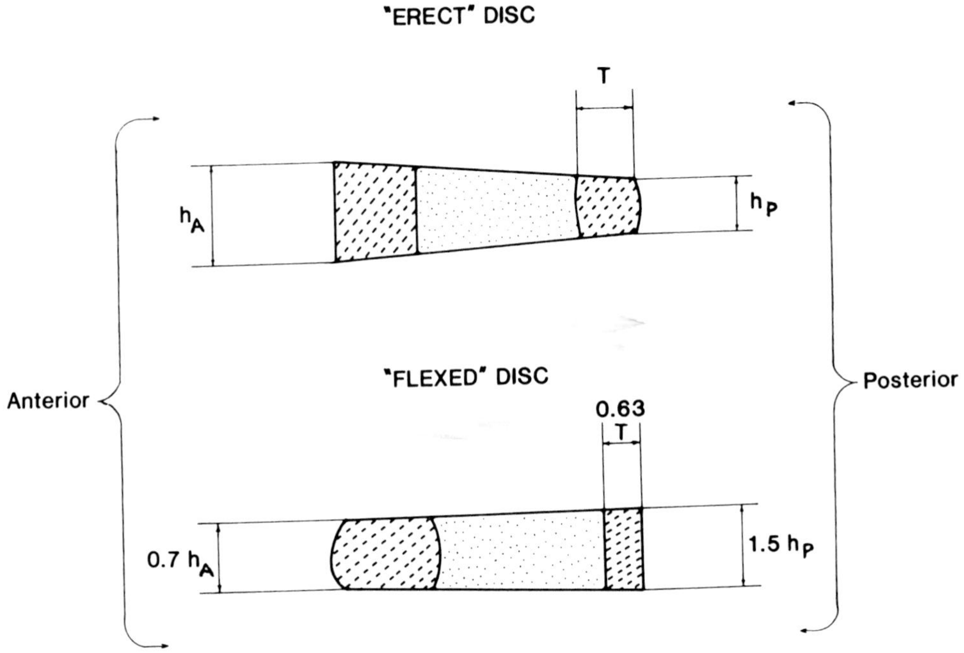

FIGURE 5. Deformation of the annulus fibrosus of lumbar discs in flexed posture as compared to erect posture. The deformation is inferred from changes in disc space height as seen on sagittal-plane X-rays of people in the erect standing and toe-touching postures.[45,46]

opposite side.[43] Thus, flexion increases the bulge anteriorly while extension increases it posteriorly.

Wedging the disc, either in flexion or extension, increases the hydrostatic pressure in the nucleus pulposus for the same applied load,[5] presumably because deforming the disc increases the prestressing of the nucleus by the fibers of the annulus. This increase in hydrostatic pressure can be considerable at low load levels, appropriate for sitting and standing, but it may not occur at all at high load levels since flexed motion segments have a high compressive strength.[6,44]

An asymmetrically compressed motion segment can fail in a number of ways. If wedged in moderate flexion, the site of failure is usually the vertebral body end-plate.[6] However, extreme wedging in hyperflexion causes failure either in the anterior wall of the vertebral body or in the posterior annulus of the disc (see Section VII).

C. Tension

Discs are rarely subjected to pure tensile forces in life. Even during traction, the muscles of the trunk can act to keep the discs compressed.

Table 4
TENSILE STRENGTH CHARACTERISTICS OF CADAVERIC INTERVERTEBRAL DISCS[31]

	Cervical discs	Thoracic discs	Lumbar discs
Tensile breaking load (N)	1030	1393—2855	3865
Tensile strength MPa	3.2	2.5	2.9
Ultimate elongation (%)	89	56	68

Note: Discs were from cadavers aged between 20 and 39 years.

Cadaveric discs have been tested to failure in tension,[31] and the results for cadavers aged between 20 and 39 years are shown in Table 4. The elastic limit was reached at about 75% of the tensile strength values given. Failure occurred by a splitting of the cartilage end-plates, or by the disc pulling a fragment of bone away from the posterior vertebral body.

V. BENDING

The ranges of the principal bending movements that occur in life and the position of the center of rotation are described in Section II.C. The mechanism by which a disc permits bending is essentially the same for flexion, lateral flexion, and extension, so only flexion will be described.

In full flexion, the disc deforms as shown in Figure 5. The reduction in height of the anterior annulus and the stretching of the posterior annulus can be inferred from changes in the disc space height seen on sagittal-plane X-rays of voluteers in the erect standing and fully flexed postures.[45,46] The changes in thickness of the annulus can be calculated from the height changes since the annular volume must remain constant. (The volume of a piece of disc tissue can only be changed if its fluid content changes, and fluid flow is so slow that it can be disregarded during a bending movement.) The thinning of the posterior annulus in full flexion has been confirmed by comparing the rate of diffusion of a radioactive tracer into flexed and erect discs.[47]

The deformation shown in Figure 5 is much greater than that which occurs in compression or axial rotation, and it cannot be accounted for simply by stretching of the collagen fibers. Probably what happens is that the obliquely running fibers of the annulus change their orientation during bending movements.[30,48] As the posture changes from erect to flexed, the radial bulging of the posterior annulus decreases, giving a small amount of slack to each fiber. Then, because of the oblique course of the fibers, this small amount of slack allows a considerable vertical separation of the end-plate, as the fiber orientation changes. The high deformability of annulus material in the vertical direction has been verified in tensile tests on small samples of tissue (Section III.A).

For the reasons discussed above, intervertebral discs offer very little resistance to the first few degrees of bending.[24,27] However, as the limit of the range of motion is approached and the fibers of the annulus become severely stretched, the bending resistance rises considerably. A lumbar disc can resist a bending moment of about 13 Nm before failure.[23] Then the fibers of the posterior annulus either tear away from their attachments or else pull a fragment of bone from the vertebral body.[46] The tension in the collagen network of a flexed disc increases the prestressing of the nucleus pulposus, causing its hydrostatic pressure to rise.[5] However, disc prolapse does not occur unless this pressure is raised even further by simultaneous compression of the disc (Section VII).

Lumbar discs resist extension more strongly than flexion or lateral flexion. Typically, a bending moment of 4.7 Nm causes about 5.9° of flexion, 4.2° of lateral flexion, and 3.6°

of extension.[27] These figures probably reflect the relative resistance to stretching of the posterior, lateral, and anterior annulus.

A disc's resistance to bending depends on the volume of the nucleus pulposus, perhaps because this determines the amount of slack in the fibers of the annulus. If the nuclear volume is increased (by saline injection) then the resistance to bending increases.[49] If it is decreased (by chemonucleolysis[50] or by creep loading[23]), then the resistance to bending falls.

VI. TORSION

The range of axial rotation that occurs in life and the position of the center of rotation are described in Section II.D. Because the collagen fibers of the annulus are oriented in two separate directions, only half of the fibers can resist clockwise rotations and the other half anticlockwise rotations. However, this does not mean that the disc is particularly weak in torsion, since the fibers that do resist a given movement are aligned to provide maximum resistance. (Annulus fibrosus material is strongest when stretched parallel to one of the two fiber directions; see Section III.A).

Discs are stiffer in torsion than in bending. Typically, a moment of 4.7 Nm will cause about 5.9° of flexion and 3.6° of extension, but a torque of 4.7 Nm will cause only 1.7° of axial rotation.[27] During axial rotation, the increasing stress in the collagen fibers raises the hydrostatic pressure in the nucleus pulposus, but this pressure increase is considerably less than that occurring in bending.[27]

When a cadaveric lumbar disc is subjected to combined torsion and compression in order to simulate twisting movements in life, the disc recovers completely from rotations of up to about 9°.[51] Beyond this limit, inelastic stretching occurs, and the disc fails completely in torsion at angles between 10° and 26°.[52] Torsional strength data[31] for discs aged 20 to 39 years are given in Table 5. At failure, the outer lamellae of the annulus become separated from each other and tear away from their vertebral attachments.[31,52] Torsion does not damage the nucleus or inner annulus, no radial fissures are formed, and the disc does not prolapse.

Despite these experimental results and despite the fact that the lumbar apophyseal joints limit axial rotation to about 1° to each side per lumbar level,[26,29,53,54] it is still widely believed that torsion can damage the lumbar discs in life. It could be argued that repeated small rotations to 1° could cause microscopic damage that is not detectable in cadaveric experiments. However, this theory is hard to reconcile with the fact that thoracic discs (which are not so well protected by the apophyseal joints) have a much greater range of axial rotation in life (see Table 1).

VII. COMPRESSION AND BENDING: DISC PROLAPSE

There have been numerous attempts to make cadaveric discs prolapse by subjecting them to high compressive forces. Compressing a disc raises the hydrostatic pressure in the nucleus pulposus, causing it to press outward on the annulus fibrosus and the vertebral end-plates (see Section IV.A). However, only annulus protrusion has occasionally been obtained in this way, and this has occurred in discs that had been allowed to swell up in saline before testing.[37] Usually, in an erect (unflexed) spine, the weak link is the end-plate, and this fractures, sometimes allowing nuclear pulp into the vertebral body.[9,41] The same thing happens when the compressive force is applied cyclically,[55,56] when the nuclear pressure is raised by fluid injection,[57] or when the annulus is first weakened by cutting into it with a scalpel.[32,58] Even when a channel is cut internally from the nucleus outward into the posterior annulus, a compressive force still fractures the end-plate.[59]

For posterior prolapse to occur, the posterior annulus must first be made weaker than the end-plate, using some physiological means. The obvious method is to wedge the disc in

Table 5
**TORSIONAL STRENGTH CHARACTERISTICS OF CADAVERIC
INTERVERTEBRAL DISCS[31]**

	Cervical discs	Thoracic discs	Lumbar discs
Breaking torsional moment (Nm)	5.5	8.5—26.8	45.4
Torsional strength (N/mm²)	5.1	4.6	5.0
Ultimate angle of torsion (°)	38	29—18	15

Note: Discs were from cadavers aged between 20 and 39 years.

flexion since this stretches and thins the posterior annulus (see Section V) while at the same time shifting compressive force off the central portion of the end-plate onto the anterior annulus (see Section IV.B). When this was tried by flexing motion segments by 4° to 8° and then compressing them to failure, the discs still would not prolapse.[6] However, the specimens were stronger than when simply compressed, and failure occurred in various parts of the vertebral body, not just the end-plates, suggesting that the weak link was being bypassed.

The solution to the problem was suggested by Rissanen's[60] work on the interspinous ligaments. He showed that they are damaged in a high proportion of cadaver spines and quoted Killanin that they were "almost invariably slack in cases of prolapsed disc brought to surgery". Now, the interspinous ligament is the first structure to be damaged when the physiological limit of flexion is exceeded (see Section II.C). Perhaps disc prolapse is caused, not by excessive compression combined with moderate flexion, but by excessive flexion with moderate compression. This hypothesis was tested in our laboratory by wedging a motion segment in hyperflexion (so that the interspinous and supraspinous ligaments were overstretched) and then rapidly compressing it. The disc prolapsed immediately.

Since then, nearly 100 disc prolapses have been obtained under controlled loading conditions. Two fundamentally different types of disc lesions occur, depending on how the compressive force is applied. A single application of load, as described above, causes a sudden prolapse, while fatigue (cyclic) loading causes a gradual prolapse. These experiments will now be described in detail in order to give an exact account of the mechanisms involved and also to indicate the difficulty of simulating physiological events on cadaveric material.

A. Sudden Prolapse

1. Method

Cadaveric motion segments were dissected free of muscle, and the contents of the spinal canal were removed with forceps. In the first 61 tests,[46] the laminae were sawed off to give an unrestricted view of the posterior annulus, but in later tests, the neural arch was left intact. Each specimen was securely held in two cups of dental plaster (Q. S. Stonehard) with the midplane of the disc parallel to the ends of the cups (Figure 6). The anteroposterior axis of the specimen was usually set at an angle of about 15° to the sides of the cups, so that the apparatus shown in Figure 6 produced a combination of lateral flexion and forward flexion, and so stressed one of the posterolateral corners of the disc more than the other.*

The angle plate was adjusted so that the specimen was flexed to the limit of its physiological range as determined by the elastic limit of the supra-/interspinous ligaments.[19] In the early tests, where the laminae were removed, this angle had to be estimated using X-ray data. While wedged in this way, the specimen was compressed by a force rising at 3000 N/sec up to a predetermined maximum load which corresponded to vigorous back muscle activity for a person of the same age and body mass as the cadaver being tested. A force deformation

---

* This was not always the case, and prolapses could be obtained without a component of lateral flexion.

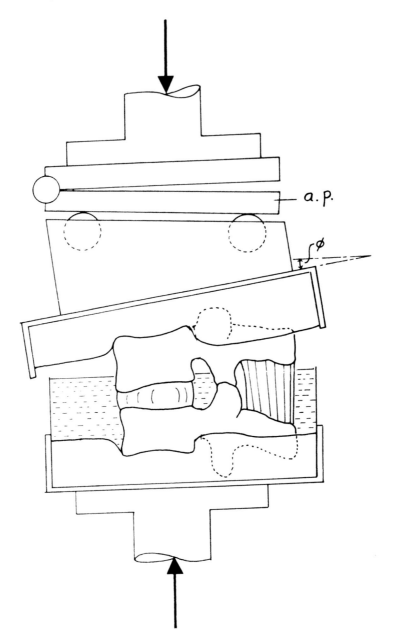

FIGURE 6.   Apparatus for testing a cadaveric motion segment in combined compression and bending. The flexion angle Ø is selected by means of a variable angle plate a.p. The specimen is surrounded by a bath of saline.

curve was plotted during loading (Figure 7, curve A). If failure of the specimen was not indicated, the flexion angle was increased by 1° or 2°, and the same load was applied again. This process was repeated at higher and higher angles until failure did occur or until it was obvious that the capsular ligaments were being torn, in which case the specimen was tested to failure at that angle. Force deformation curves were drawn whenever the disc was flexed to higher angles, to check that it was not damaged by the bending moment. If it was, the test was abandoned.

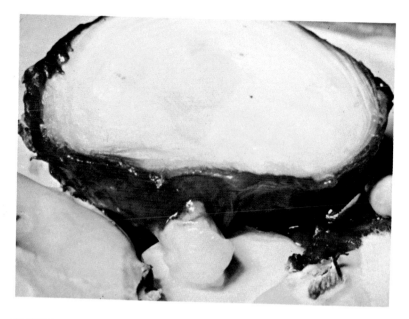

PLATE 1. A sudden prolapse simulated on a cadaveric disc. Note that the disc shows no sign of degeneration. Compare Figure 8. (From Adams, M. A. and Hutton, W. C., *Spine*, 7 (3), 189, 1982. With permission.)

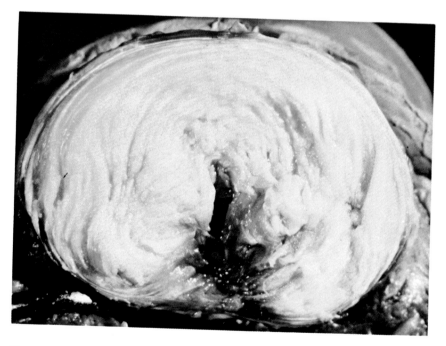

PLATE 2. A sudden prolapse simulated on a cadaveric disc. This is an annular protusion. See Figure 9.

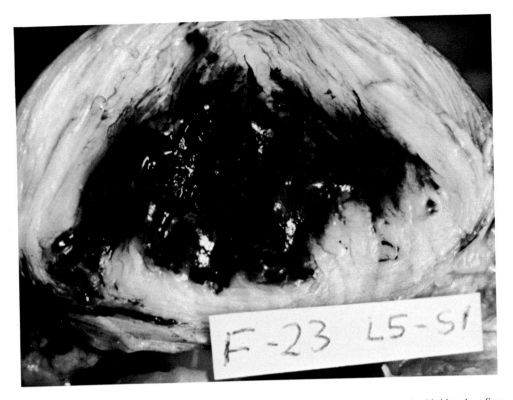

PLATE 3.   A gradual prolapse simulated on a cadaveric disc. The nuclear pulp is stained with blue dye. See Figure 11. (From Adams, M. A. and Hutton, W. C., *J. Bone Jt. Surg.*, 65-B (2), 201, 1983. With permission.)

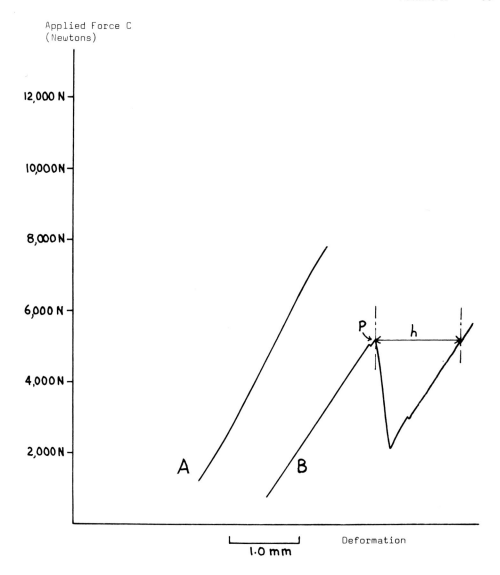

FIGURE 7. Force deformation curves for a motion segment compressed as shown in Figure 6. At low flexion angles (curve A) the specimen is not damaged; but at high flexion angles (curve B) the intervertebral disc can prolapse, and then the specimen suddenly loses height (h). (From Adams, M. A. and Hutton, W. C., *Spine*, 7(3), 188, 1982. With permission.)

2. Results

In the original series of 61 tests, 26 of the motion segments failed by a posterior prolapse of the intervertebral discs; the other 35 specimens sustained vertebral fractures of various kinds. (A similar striking rate was found in subsequent experiments, but many of these were performed under slightly different conditions from those described. For simplicity, the results from the original series only are presented here.)

A typical load deformation curve for a specimen failing by disc prolapse is curve B in Figure 7. The prolapse (point P) causes a sudden reduction in disc volume, but because there is no bone damage and the annulus is largely intact, the stiffness of the motion segment is little impaired and the gradient of the graph after prolapse is similar to that before. The reduction in disc height caused by prolapse (h in Figure 7) was 0.7 mm on average with a maximum of 1.3 mm.

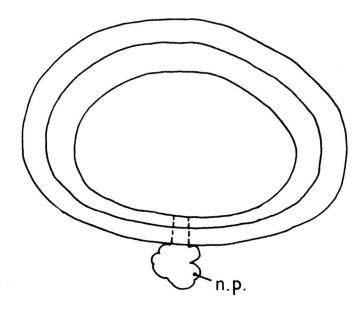

FIGURE 8.   A sudden prolapse simulated on a cadaveric disc (n.p. = nucleus pulposus). Compare Plate 1. (From Adams, M. A. and Hutton, W. C., *Spine*, 7(3), 189, 1982. With permission.)

A typical prolapse is shown in Figure 8 and Plate 1.* This is a nuclear extrusion with nuclear pulp having burst through a channel in the annulus to lie outside the disc. In most cases, the channel lay adjacent to one of the cartilage end-plates. They have remarkably good self-sealing properties and would not permit any pulp to be pushed back into the discs. Occasionally, it was found that manipulating the specimen (pulling the vertebrae apart, and bending the specimen in flexion) would cause the pulp to be sucked back in again, though it invariably reappeared when the traction was released. The word channel has been used to denote the hole punched through the annulus, because the more usual term, "fissure," implies a widespread distortion of the lamellae of the annulus and a migration of nuclear material toward the disc periphery. Sudden prolapse caused no such distortion. In fact, the bisected discs looked perfectly normal. The extruded nuclear pulp appeared either centrally or on the posterolateral corner which was more heavily stressed by the component of lateral bending. Large central extrusions ruptured the posterior longitudinal ligament, whereas smaller extrusions either formed a bulge behind it (giving the impression of a protruding annulus) or were deflected sideways to one or both posterolateral corners. The consistency of the extruded material varied from stringy in a 53-year-old, to soft in a 30-year-old, while from a 14-year-old disc it resembled a viscous, translucent fluid that flowed under its own weight. In cases of nuclear extrusion, the vertebral end-plates were undamaged, and no blood was expressed from the vertebral body.

Eight of the 26 prolapses took a different form from that described above; they were annular protrusions. In these discs the midline posterior annulus was soft and bulged slightly into the spinal canal and was usually stained with blood (Figure 9 and Plate 2*). There was a more or less distinct fissure from the nucleus, but no nuclear material was expressed through it. The outermost lamella of the annulus, with the adhering posterior longitudinal ligament, appeared to be overstretched and slack, though its attachment to the vertebrae remained sound. The vertebral end-plates were not damaged, but blood was expressed from

* Plate 1 follows page 54.
* Plate 2 follows page 54.

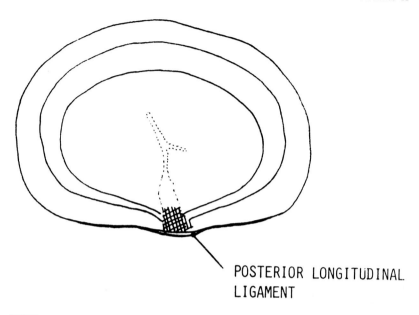

POSTERIOR LONGITUDINAL
LIGAMENT

FIGURE 9.   Diagram of sudden prolapse simulated on a cadaveric disc. This is an annular protrusion. See Plate 2.

the vertebral bodies either anteriorly or into the spinal canal. These annular protrusions were somewhat problematical; they could best be described as a localized collapse of the midline posterior annulus.

The average compressive force required to produce sudden prolapse was 5448 N (range, 2760 N to 12,968 N), and the average flexion angle was 15.8° (range, 9° to 21°). When this experiment was first reported, the flexion angles given were all 3° too low. This was because of a zero error in the scale used to measure the relative positions of the two rollers (see Figure 6). Table 6 shows how the likelihood of a disc prolapsing depends on its spinal level, age, and stage of degeneration. The most striking feature of this table is that it disproves the notion that only degenerated discs can prolapse. The mechanism of sudden prolapse is depicted in Figure 10.

B. Gradual Prolapse
1. Method

Cadaveric motion segments from subjects aged between 8 and 53 years were dissected and set in cups of plaster as described above. The neural arch and ligaments were left intact. During the fatigue testing period, the specimen was surrounded by a bath of Ringer's solution to prevent dehydration. (A humidity chamber may not be adequate for this task. Surrounding the disc by saturated water vapor prevents disc dehydration by evaporation, but it is necessary to surround the disc with water in the liquid phase if the disc's swelling pressure is to operate, as in life, to reduce the outflow of fluid caused by loading.)

As before, each specimen was wedged in forward and lateral flexion and then compressed, but this time the compressive force oscillated sinusoidally between high and low values 40 times per minute. Several slight variations in testing procedures were used.[61,62] The one that proved most successful in producing gradual prolapse was as follows.

One hour before fatigue loading commenced, the disc to be tested was injected with about 0.6 mℓ of radiopaque fluid (Conray 480) containing a few drops of blue dye (aniline blue). The needle was inserted anteriorly so that it would not damage the posterior annulus. Discograms were taken in the sagittal and coronal planes to determine the size and position

Table 6
EFFECT OF DISC DEGENERATION, AGE, AND SPINAL LEVEL ON THE LIKELIHOOD OF SUDDEN PROLAPSE

	Degree of disc degeneration				Age of cadaver (years)					Spinal level				
	1	2	3	4	<30	30—39	40—49	50—59	>59	L5—S1	L4—5	L3—4	L2—3	L1—2
No. specimens tested	15	17	24	5	16	14	9	14	8	19	12	13	9	8
% Failing by prolapsed intervertebral disc	33	71	38	0	31	50	78	50	0	53	50	31	33	38

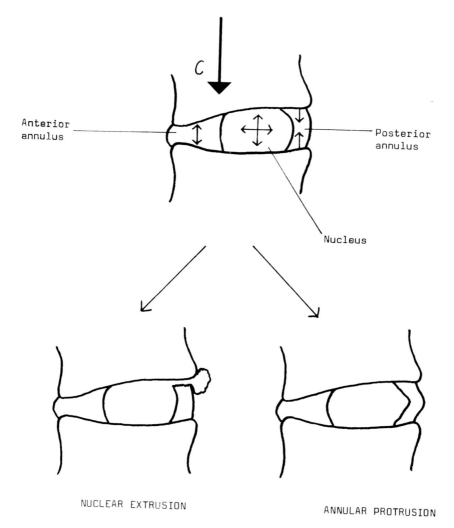

FIGURE 10.   The mechanism of sudden prolapse. Hyperflexion stretches and thins the posterior annulus, making it the weakest structure surrounding the nucleus. A high compressive force C then raises the hydrostatic pressure in the nucleus until it either bursts through the posterior annulus or causes it to collapse outward.

of the nucleus prior to testing and to demonstrate that the disc was not already fissured. (If it was, it was not tested.)

Fatigue loading began with the specimen flexed to a moderate angle, well within the physiological range and with a peak compressive force of about 1000 N to 2000 N. After 1 hr it was always found that the disc and ligaments had adapted to the wedging angle, so the specimen was flexed an extra 1° without exceeding the elastic range of these tissues. This process was repeated several times, at 1-hr intervals, until the flexion angles were higher than the normal limit of flexion expected for that specimen. Eventually, the flexion angle could not be further increased without risk of damaging the specimen. This final wedging angle was kept for the rest of the test. Its value ranged from 8° to 19°.

With the flexion angle fixed, the peak compressive force was then increased by increments of 500 N at half-hourly intervals until failure occurred. This ensured that each specimen was tested for at least half an hour (1200 cycles) at a load near its physiological limit.

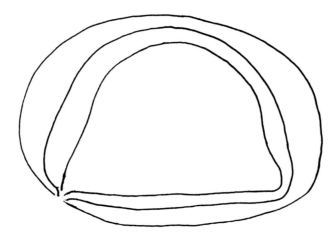

FIGURE 11.   A gradual prolapse simulated on a cadaveric disc. Compare Plate 3. (From Adams, M. A. and Hutton, W. C., *J. Bone Jt. Surg.*, 65-B(2), 201, 1983. With permission.)

2. Results

The average value of the peak compressive force at failure was 3800 N. The average duration of each test was $5^{1}/_{2}$ hr. Of 29 specimens tested in this way, 23 sustained vertebral fractures of the end-plate or anterior wall, but in 6 specimens there was a gradual prolapse of the intervertebral disc.

Blue-stained nuclear pulp first appeared underneath the surface of the annulus. In five cases, the pulp appeared at the posterolateral corner that was being more highly stressed, and in the other it appeared centrally. Over the course of a few hundred loading cycles, the pulp worked its way to the surface and oozed out. In one specimen a considerable amount of soft pulp was extruded and flowed down onto the pedicle. However, in the others only a very small quantity could be driven out, even when the compressive force was increased until the vertebrae were crushed.

"Before" and "after" discograms confirmed that a radial fissure had been formed during the testing period, and this could clearly be seen when the discs were bisected (Figure 11 and Plate 3*). The lamellae of the annulus appeared distorted into a bell shape, being closely packed anteriorly, widely spaced laterally, and tightly curved and packed in the posterolateral corners. Many of the discs which did not prolapse showed a similar pattern of annular distortion, but the nucleus had not quite managed to break through the tightly packed lamellae at the end of the fissure. The toughness of this final barrier was illustrated in two tests. When it became obvious that the vertebrae were crumbling without the disc protruding, the outermost $1^{1}/_{2}$ mm of annulus was cut away, and in both cases there was an immediate large prolapse, similar to that shown in Figure 8.

All six gradual prolapses occurred in motion segments at the L4—5 and L5—51 levels, and in each case the disc was not degenerated. The ages of the specimens were 15, 23, 23, 28, 34, and 44 years.

The mechanism of gradual prolapse is probably as shown in Figure 12. There is an outward radial pressure P on the annulus due to compression of the fluid nucleus and on anteroposterior pressure gradient G due to the flexion angle. Adding the components together gives the resultant pressure acting as shown on three points of a typical lamella. Fluid in the disc attempts to flow from high to low pressure but is obstructed by the proteoglycan gel, which in turn is obstructed by the collagen network. Consequently the lamellae are deformed along

* Plate 3 follows page 54.

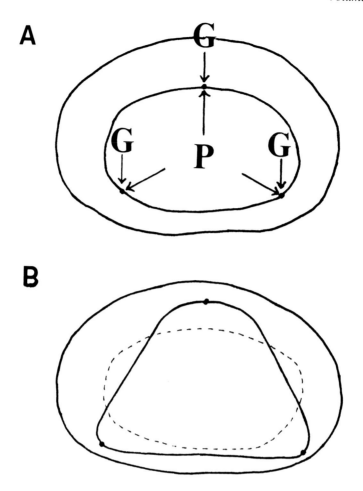

FIGURE 12. The mechanism of gradual prolapse. P, outward radial pressure; G, pressure gradient; A, before cyclic loading; B, after cyclic loading. See the text for details.

the lines of the resultant pressure gradient to form posterolateral radial fissures. Eventually nuclear pulp breaks through the distorted lamellae and escapes from the disc. Radial fissure formation requires the redistribution of fluid within the disc, and as this is a slow, time-dependent process, radial fissures are not formed when discs prolapse suddenly.

C. Disc Prolapse in Life

First, we will consider whether there is anything that might prevent the discs of living people from prolapsing by the two methods described above. Second, we will weigh the evidence that, in life, discs not only can, but do prolapse like this.

There should be no fundamental objection to applying the results of mechanical tests on cadaveric discs to living people. Since disc tissue is avascular, its mechanical properties are unlikely to change immediately after death, and it has been reported that they do not change significantly after freezing and thawing.[4,30]

These tests were performed at 21°C, but this would have made prolapses harder to achieve, since at body temperature the nucleus pulposus would have been less viscous and so more capable of breaking through the posterior annulus.

As far as the sudden prolapses are concerned, the compressive forces used (5400 N on average) are well within the scope of the back muscles during heavy lifting.[6] In some cases prolapse occurred at loads as low as 2800 N, and this force could be generated simply by picking a book off the floor. By contrast, the flexion angles used were decidedly beyond the normal physiological range, but this is no drawback. If sudden prolapse occurred at normal loads and normal flexion angles, we would all suffer the injury. Hyperflexion might occur during a rapid or uncoordinated bending movement or in a fall, in which case sudden prolapse would be accompanied by ligament injury, as suggested by Rissanen.[60] Alternatively, hyperflexion might occur as a creep process during sustained bending since, under constant tension, the ligaments and disc slowly deform as fluid is expressed from the tissues. This can result in extra flexion[23,63] even though the fluid movement, and hence creep, are reversible and the tissues are undamaged. Another possibility is that, in life, sudden prolapse can occur at lower flexion angles in a disc that has already been severely weakened by fatigue.

Let us now consider the chances of a gradual prolapse in life. In the fatigue tests, neither the flexion angles nor the peak compressive forces exceeded the physiological limits, but the relentless nature of the loading (2400 cycles/hr for up to 8 hr) plainly represents the worst job you ever had! The intention in these tests was to condense several days', or even weeks', work into one afternoon, and this can only be justified if the repair processes in life have no effect over days or weeks. As far as cellular processes are concerned, this is a reasonable assumption, since proteoglycan turnover time is 2 to 3 years[64] and for collagen it is probably even longer.[65] However, there is a physical repair mechanism that cannot be ignored: diurnal flow of fluid into and out of the disc (see Section X.A) may well retard the formation of radial fissures. The bell-shaped deformation of the lamellae of the annulus shown in Figure 11 is not an elastic deformation that disappears as soon as the deforming stress is removed. It is a permanent set involving the redistribution of fluid in the disc. For this reason, the deformation process will be hindered by diurnal fluid flow. This does not mean that the mechanism of gradual prolapse will not happen in life as in the experiment, but the time scale will be changed from hours to days or even years.

Injecting a small quantity of fluid into the nucleus pulposus before testing has a negligible effect on the outcome of the gradual prolapse tests. The fluid is quickly incorporated into the proteoglycan-water gel,[33] and by the time prolapse occurs, the water content of this gel is probably lower than before the injection.[62] Besides, the same process of radial fissure formation can be demonstrated without injecting fluid into the disc.[61]

Thus, there is no good reason why discs should not prolapse in life as in the experiments, but do they? There is plenty of epidemiological and clinical evidence linking acute low back pain and sciatica with forward bending and lifting.[66,67] There is also the pathological evidence referred to above, showing that posterior ligament injuries are common and associated with disc prolapse.[60]

On the other hand, there is no strong correlation between occupation and the incidence of disc prolapse,[68] and often prolapse is not associated with any mechanical incident recalled by the patient. The first point can be easily dealt with: people who survive in heavy manual jobs have, or soon acquire, strong backs. Muscle hypertrophy will be accompanied by bone hypertrophy and, in the long term, disc hypertrophy. It is possible that an office worker with a weak spine would be more at risk of a sudden prolapse in his leisure pursuits than a manual worker, though less at risk of a gradual prolapse. As for the second point, the lack of any mechanical incident prior to prolapse, this suggests that fatigue loading or biochemical degenerative processes (or both) leave a disc so vulnerable that it prolapses under low loads. This possibility is represented by the diagonal line in Figure 13, which is an attempt to summarize the etiology of prolapsed intervertebral disc.

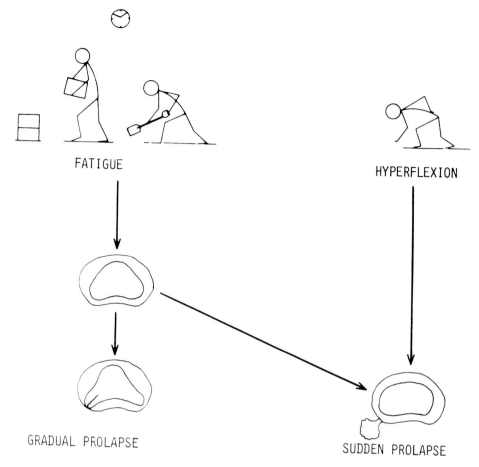

FIGURE 13. The etiology of prolapsed intervertebral disc as suggested by the results of experiments on cadaveric discs.

VIII. TIME-DEPENDENT MECHANICAL PROPERTIES

Some of the most interesting mechanical properties of the disc are time dependent; that is, they depend on how rapidly a force is applied or for how long it is applied. The main cause of this time-dependent behavior is fluid flow within the proteoglycan-water gel of the matrix.

A. Fluid Flow

The water content of the gel is variable and represents an equilibrium between two opposing pressures: mechanical pressure acting on the disc, which dehydrates the gel; and the swelling pressure of the hydrophilic proteoglycans, which causes the gel to absorb fluid. Any change in the loading of the disc disturbs this equilibrium, and fluid flows until a new balance is achieved.

The process is very slow because of high internal resistance to the movement of water molecules in the gel. Experiments on cadaveric lumbar discs show that 24 hr of loading at 981 N reduces the water content of the nucleus and annulus by 8% and 11%, respectively.[69] The amount of fluid flow that occurs during various activities in life and its effect on metabolite transport are considered in Section X.A.

The water expelled during loading is reabsorbed when the load is removed. Calculations

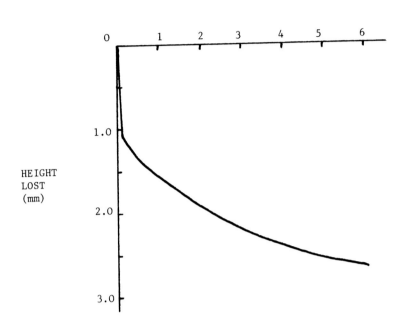

FIGURE 14.   Disc creep. When a lumbar motion segment is loaded in compression (1000 N in this case) the intervertebral disc loses height. The initial, almost instantaneous deformation is termed elastic and the subsequent slow deformation is called creep.

show that water expelled over a period of 16 hr can be recovered in just 8 hr, provided the disc is immersed in saline.[70] If it is not immersed, then recovery will take longer[71] or be incomplete.[58]

Axial loading probably causes fluid to flow radially outward from the disc,[72] and fluid loss is then a maximum in the annulus and a minimum in the nucleus.[69,73] Eccentric loading, however, creates nonradial pressure gradients in the disc,[35] resulting in a different redistribution of the water of the disc. For example, flexing a disc creates an anterior-posterior pressure gradient, and if this is maintained for several hours, the resulting fluid flow can leave the disc wedged in slight flexion even when the load is removed.[63] (It is likely that the original fluid distribution and hence disc shape would be regained in time.) A combination of compression and flexion causes both radial and anterior-posterior pressure gradients, and this can explain the formation of radial fissures in discs (see Section VII.B).

B. Creep

If a constant load is applied to a disc, it loses height, as shown in Figure 14. The initial, almost instantaneous, deformation is termed elastic because it is reversed if the load is removed promptly. However, if the load is not removed, the disc continues to deform, rapidly at first but more slowly later. This is creep, and the creep deformation is recovered slowly when the load is removed. Creep deformation involves height loss, as shown in Figure 14, and also increased radial bulging of the disc.[71]

The underlying cause of creep is fluid flow, and the mechanisms are probably as follows. First, fluid loss reduces the volume and hence the height of a disc. Second, a reduced nuclear volume gives more slack to the fibers of the annulus and allows it to bulge outward like a flat tire.[34,37] At load levels corresponding to standing and sitting postures, most of the height loss is probably due to volume reduction,[73] while at higher load levels and after longer periods of creep, annulus deformation becomes more important.[71] It is possible that creep stretching of the collagen fibers of the annulus may contribute to annular bulging,[71] but this has not been proven.

Creep changes the mechanical characteristics of the discs. After creep, a disc is stiffer in compression,[71] and it behaves more elastically in the sense that it recovers more rapidly from further deformations and dissipates less energy during a loading-unloading cycle.[58,71] However, this does not mean that its function as a shock absorber is in any way impaired, since shocks (or accelerations) can be damped by purely elastic deformations (as in a bedspring, for example). In fact, reducing the water content (and volume) of the nucleus makes the disc better adapted to withstand high compressive forces, because the nucleus is then less likely to prolapse through the posterior annulus.[23] Creep reduces the resistance of a disc to bending and increases its range of flexion.[23]

These effects, like the extra radial bulging, can be attributed to increased slack in the fibers of the annulus. A corollary of this is that resistance to bending is increased[49] and radial bulging decreased[34] when disc height is artificially raised by means of a saline injection into the nucleus. Similar creep effects can be caused by repeated tensile testing of annulus slices.[30] The process is essentially the same: the fluid content of the tissue is reduced, leaving it stiffer and more elastic.

Disc creep affects the mechanics of the whole spine because it brings the vertebrae closer together. The lumbar apophyseal joints (and, in rare cases, the spinous processes) then resist part of the compressive force on the spine.[11,12] The intervertebral ligaments gain some slack and allow more flexion.[23] Conversely, the ranges of extension and axial rotation are probably reduced because these movements are limited by bony contact between the neural arches.[51]

C. Effect of Loading Rate on Disc Mechanics

This has not been thoroughly investigated. It might be expected that discs would resist rapidly applied loads more vigorously than slowly applied ones, since rapid loading does not give the water any time to get out of the way. Unpublished results from our own laboratory show that a motion segment is stiffer when compressed rapidly. Tensile tests on slices of annulus show them to have better elastic recovery when stretched rapidly.[30]

IX. VARIATIONS WITH AGE AND SPINAL LEVEL

Cadaveric discs show considerable variation in mechanical properties. Much of this variation can be attributed to the size of the discs (for example, a large disc will deform less than a small disc if the same force is applied to it), and this explains the observed differences between male and female discs.[38] However, certain morphological and mechanical properties show consistent variations with age and spinal level.

A. Age

With increasing age, discs show a regular increase in macroscopically observable degenerative changes.[74] The average water content decreases from about 78% at age 15 to 65% at age 80,[73,74] with most of the reduction occurring in the nucleus.[69,73] Between the ages of 20 and 60, the height of a typical thoracic disc decreases from 7 mm to 4 mm, and that of a typical lumbar disc decreases from 10 mm to 8 $\frac{1}{2}$ mm.[74] The cross-sectional area increases during childhood, stays roughly constant between the ages of 20 and 60, and then increases again in certain old discs,[74] perhaps as a result of remodeling of the vertebral body. The axial deformability of adult discs shows little age dependence,[74] but small samples of annulus fibrosus become more extensible and less elastic in degenerated (presumably older) discs.[30] This latter property may explain why old degenerated discs bulge more under load[42] and why old discs creep more rapidly than young discs[74,75] even though they lose less water in the process.[73]

Little is known about age-related changes in the bending and torsional properties of discs since, in experiments on motion segments, these are masked by age-related changes in the intervertebral ligaments and apophyseal joints. However, isolated discs aged between 40 and 70 years were found to have an average tensile strength 25% lower than discs aged 20 to 40 years.[31]

B. Spinal Level

The orientation of collagen fibers in the annulus is the same in all regions of the spine,[76] and the average water content of the discs does not vary significantly between T5—6 and L5—S1.[77] However, there are morphological changes in the discs at different levels. Average disc height increases regularly from about 3 mm at T5—6 to 11 mm at L4—5, while cross-sectional area increases from about 6 cm^2 at T5—6 to 16 cm^2 at L4—5.[77]

The increase in disc height explains why axial deformability and radial bulging increase down the spine for the same applied compressive force.[77] High discs probably creep more, but this can be masked in cadaveric experiments if the applied compressive force is not kept proportional to the cross-sectional area of the discs.

The greater height and the wedge shape of the L4—5 and L5—S1 discs probably contribute to the increase sagittal mobility of the lower lumbar spine (Table 1). The relative strengths of cervical, thoracic, and lumbar discs are shown in Tables 3, 4, and 5.

X. MECHANICAL FACTORS IN DISC NUTRITION

The intervertebral discs are the largest avascular structures in the body. Nutrients reach the chondrocytes in the disc by two routes: (1) from the blood vessels in the vertebral body, through the central, permeable part of the vertebral end-plate; and (2) from the blood vessels and tissue fluid surrounding the annulus fibrosus. The transport processes are fluid flow and diffusion. Fluid flow, caused by pressure changes on the disc (see Section VIII.A), is effective in transporting large molecules such as proteins,[78] while diffusion is more effective for small molecules.[79] Both of these transport processes are affected by long-term or postural loading of the disc.

In what follows, postures are classified as erect if they preserve or increase the lumbar lordosis and as flexed if they flatten the lumbar lordosis. Typical erect and flexed postures are shown in Figure 15.

A. Fluid Pumping

Changes in the mechanical load acting on the spine cause fluid to flow into and out of the discs, and this fluid pumping can aid the transport of disc metabolites. The most profound change is the diurnal variation between daily activity and nightime rest. Loading that simulates a day's activity causes cadaveric lumbar discs to lose 8% of the water from the nucleus and 11% from the annulus[69] with most of this change occurring during the first 4 hr of loading.[73] This fluid exchange is affected by posture, as shown in Figure 16a. Flexed postures expel more fluid from the lumbar discs than do erect postures, with the effect being particularly marked in the nucleus.[73] Calculations show that fluid flow on this scale can improve the discs supply of glucose by a small amount,[73] but the effect on large molecules may be considerable since they diffuse much more slowly. So flexed postures can improve the fluid flow component of the metabolite transport of the discs, at least in the lumbar region. There may be similar benefits from flattening the curvature of the cervical spine.

Fluid flow can be affected by another kind of postural variation: that is, change between vigorous activity and relative inactivity. Fluid flow from the discs of living people can be inferred from accurate measurements of changes in body height.[80,81] Such measurements show that just 4 min spent lifting a heavy weight up and down can cause a height loss (and

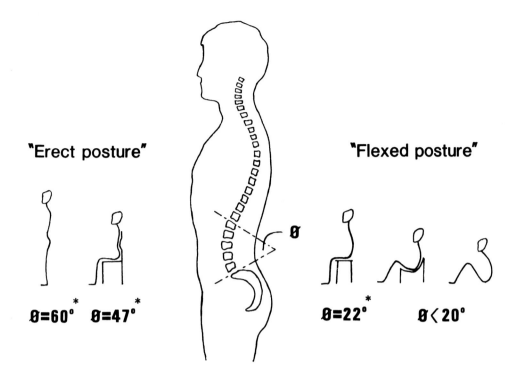

"Erect posture"

"Flexed posture"

ø=60°* ø=47°*

ø=22°* ø<20°

FIGURE 15. The lumbar curvature (Ø) is defined as the angle between the upper surfaces of the sacrum and the L1 vertebral body. Values of Ø are shown for typical erect and flexed postures. (*Calculated from Andersson et al.[86]). (From Adams, M. A. and Hutton, W. C., *J. Bone Jt. Surg.*, 67-B, 625, 1985. With permission.)

presumably a fluid loss) half as great as the diurnal variation,[81] and this height (fluid) loss is recovered after about 6 min of lying supine. Evidently, alternating vigorous activity with periods of rest can improve the fluid flow component of disc metabolite transport. The more rapid the loading fluctuations become, the more the fluid exchange is concentrated in the peripheral regions of the disc. Thus, the fluid pumping that occurs during the walking cycle has only a small effect on metabolite transport, according to calculations[70] and some experiments on dogs.[82]

B. Effect of Disc Deformation on Diffusion

Diffusion occurs as a result of a chemical concentration gradient, so nutrients diffuse into the disc and waste products diffuse out of it. Mechanical loading can affect this process by deforming the disc and altering the diffusion path length to various locations within the disc. The shorter the path length, the more rapid the metabolite transport becomes. The greatest disc deformation occurs in flexion and extension movements (see Section V), so it is not surprising that diffusion into the disc is markedly different in flexed and erect postures. This was studied by loading cadaveric lumbar motion segments to simulate either flexed or erect posture and then allowing a radioactive tracer to diffuse into the deformed discs.[47] The results are shown in Figure 16b. In erect postures, diffusion occurs more readily into the anterior annulus than into the posterior annulus, probably because the disc height decreases from front to back. Flexed postures reverse this imbalance and increase the overall rate of diffusion into the disc. The effect on the posterior annulus can be explained by assuming that it is stretched by 50% and thinned by 33% in flexed, as compared to erect, posture. This is in agreement with changes in disc space height seen on X-rays of people in the erect standing and toe-touching postures.[45,46]

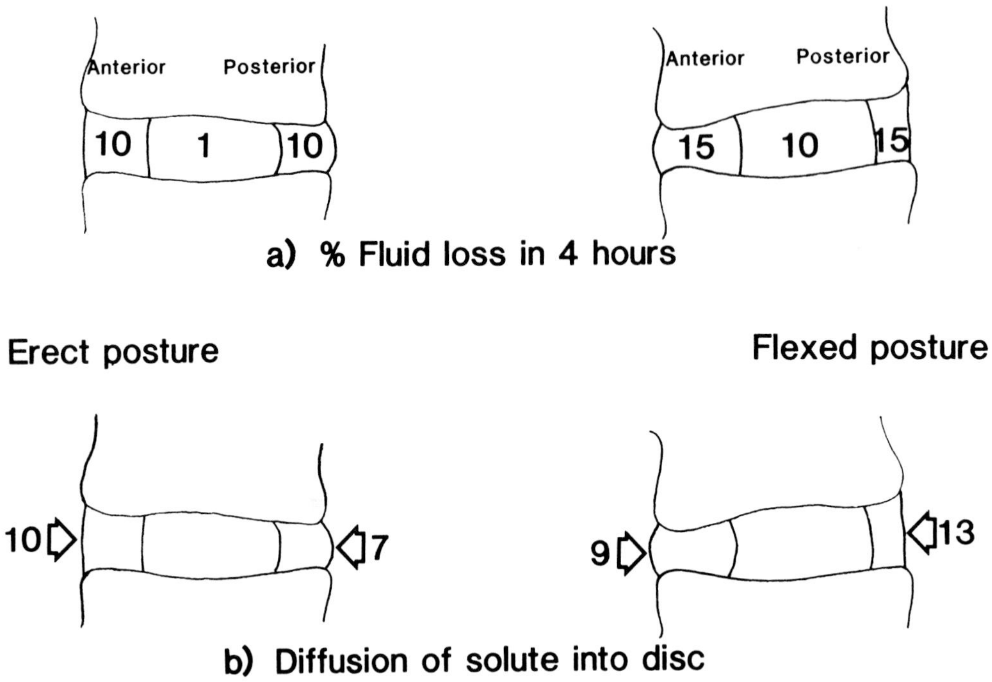

a) % Fluid loss in 4 hours

Erect posture   Flexed posture

b) Diffusion of solute into disc

FIGURE 16.   (a)Fluid loss from the disc depends on posture. The three values for each disc refer to the anterior annulus, the nucleus, and the posterior annulus. (b) In erect posture, solutes can diffuse more easily into the anterior half of the disc than into the posterior half. The imbalance is reversed in flexed posture. The numbers are proportional to the amount of solute that can diffuse in during 4 hr. (From Adams, M. A. and Hutton, W. C., *J. Bone Jt. Surg.*, 67-B(4), 627, 1985. With permission.)

To a certain extent, the increased diffusion into the posterior half of flexed discs via the annulus will be offset by a slight decrease in diffusion by the end-plate route, which was effectively shut off in the above experiment. The two effects may cancel in the posterior half of the nucleus, but there is little doubt that flexed posture increases diffusion into the inner posterior annulus, and this is precisely the part of the disc that has the least satisfactory nutrient supply in erect posture.[83] Consequently, it would seem advantageous to alternate erect posture (which is often unavoidable) with sitting postures that flex the lumbar spine.

The same conclusion may be applicable to the cervical spine, while the thoracic discs may similarly benefit from a straightening of the normal thoracic kyphosis.

C. Other Mechanisms

Mechanical factors may influence disc nutrition in other ways. For example, high pressures may directly affect the chondrocytes; postural variation and activity may affect the blood supply to the various regions of the spine; and deformations of the vertebral end-plate may hinder metabolite transport into the nucleus. Also, structural changes in the discs and end-plates caused by injury or fatigue may disrupt the nutrient pathways and adversely affect disc nutrition. None of these possibilities has been tested by experiment, and the limited data on which the above conclusions were based should be borne in mind.

REFERENCES

1. **Nachemson, A.,** Electromyographic studies on the vertebral portion of the psoas muscle, *Acta Orthop. Scand.*, 37, 177, 1966.
2. **Nachemson, A.,** Disc pressure measurements, *Spine*, 6, 93, 1981.
3. **Quinnell, R. C., Stockdale, H. R., and Willis, D. S.,** Observations of pressures within normal discs in the lumbar spine, *Spine*, 8, 166, 1983.
4. **Nachemson, A. L.,** Lumbar intradiscal pressure, *Acta Orthop.* Scand., Suppl. 43, 1960.
5. **Nachemson, A. L.,** The influence of spinal movements on the lumbar intradiscal pressure and on the tensile stresses in the annulus fibrosus, *Acta Orthop. Scand.*, 33, 183, 1963.
6. **Hutton, W. C. and Adams, M. A.,** Can the lumbar spine be crushed in heavy lifting?, *Spine*, 7, 309, 1982.
7. **Bartelink, D. L.,** The role of abdominal pressure in relieving the pressure on the lumbar intervertebral disc, *J. Bone Jt. Surg.*, 39-B, 718, 1957.
8. **Morris, J. M., Lucas, D. B., and Bresler, B.,** Role of the trunk in stability of the spine, *J. Bone Jt. Surg.*, 43-A, 327, 1961.
9. **Eie, N.,** Load capacity of the low back, *J. Oslo City Hosp.*, 16, 73, 1966.
10. **Eie, N.,** Recent measurements of the intra-abdominal pressure, in *Perspectives in Biomedical Engineering*, Kenedi, R.M., Ed., Macmillan, London, 1973, 121.
11. **Adams, M. A. and Hutton, W. C.,** The effect of posture on the role of the apophyseal joints in resisting intervertebral compressive forces, *J. Bone Jt. Surg.*, 62-B, 358, 1980.
12. **Dunlop, R. B., Adams, M. A., and Hutton, W. C.,** Disc space narrowing and the lumbar facet joints, *J. Bone Jt. Surg.*, 66-B, 706, 1984.
13. **Hutton, W. C., Stott, J. R. R., and Cyron, B. M.,** Is spondylolysis a fatigue fracture?, *Spine*, 2, 202, 1977.
14. **Cyron, B. M., Hutton, W. C., and Stott, J. R. R.,** Spondylolysis — the shearing stiffness of the lumbar intervertebral joint, *Acta Orthop. Belg.*, 45, 459, 1980.
15. **Cyron, B. M. and Hutton, W. C.,** The behaviour of the lumbar intervertebral disc under repetitive forces, *Int. Orthop.*, 5, 203, 1981.
16. **Jonck, L. M. and VanNiekerk, J. M.,** A roentgenological study of the motion of the lumbar spine of the Bantu, *S. Afr. J. Lab. Clin. Med.*, 7, 67, 1961.
17. **Taylor, J. and Twomey, L.,** Sagittal and horizontal plane movement of the human lumbar vertebral column in cadavers and in the living, *Rheumatol. Rehabil.*, 19, 223, 1980.
18. **Pearcy, M., Portek, I., and Shepherd, J.,** The effect of low back pain on lumbar spinal movements measured by three-dimensional X-ray analysis, *Spine*, 10, 150, 1985.
19. **Adams, M. A., Hutton, W. C., and Stott, J. R. R.,** The resistance to flexion of the lumbar intervertebral joint, *Spine*, 5, 245, 1980.
20. **Twomey, L. T. and Taylor, J. R.,** Sagittal movements of the human lumbar vertebral column: a quantitative study of the role of the posterior vertebral elements, *Arch. Phys. Med. Rehabil.*, 64, 322, 1983.
21. **Adams, M. A. and Hutton, W. C.,** Has the lumbar spine a margin of safety in forward bending?, *Clin. Biomech.*, 1, 3, 1986.
22. **Adams, M. A.,** The Mechanical Properties of Lumbar Intervertebral Joints with Special Reference to the Causes of Low Back Pain, Ph.D. thesis, Polytechnic of Central London, England, 1980.
23. **Adams, M. A., Dolan, P., and Hutton, W. C.,** Diurnal variations in the stresses on the lumbar spine, *Spine*, 12, 130, 1987.
24. **Markolf, K. L.,** Deformation of the thoracolumbar intervertebral joints in response to external loads, *J. Bone Jt. Surg.*, 54-A, 511, 1972.
25. **Panjabi, M. M., Krag, M. H., White, A. A., and Southwick, W. O.,** Effects of preload on load displacement curves of the lumbar spine, *Orthop. Clin. N. Am.*, 8, 181, 1977.
26. **Pearcy, M. J. and Tibrewal, S. B.,** Axial rotation and lateral bending in the normal lumbar spine measured by three-dimensional radiography, *Spine*, 9, 582, 1984.
27. **Schultz, A. B., Warwick, D. N., Berkson, M. H., and Nachemson, A. L.,** Mechanical properties of human lumbar spine segments. I. Response in flexion, extension, lateral bending and torsion, *J. Biomech. Eng.*, 101, 46, 1979.
28. **Cossette, J. W., Farfan, H. F., Robertson, G. H., and Wells, R. V.,** The instantaneous centre of rotation of the third lumbar intervertebral joint, *J. Biomech.*, 4, 149, 1971.
29. **Adams, M. A. and Hutton, W. C.,** The relevance of torsion to the mechanical derangement of the lumbar spine, *Spine*, 6, 241, 1981.
30. **Galante, J. O.,** Tensile properties of the human lumbar annulus fibrosus, *Acta Orthop. Scand.*, Suppl. 100, 1967.
31. **Sonoda, T.,** Studies on the strength for compression, tension and torsion of the human vertebral column, *J. Kyoto Pref. Med. Univ.*, 71, 659, 1962.

32. **Markolf, K. L. and Morris, J. M.,** The structural components of the intervertebral disc, *J. Bone Jt. Surg.*, 56-A, 675, 1974.

33. **Adams, M. A., Dolan, P., and Hutton, W. C.,** The stages of disc degeneration as revealed by discograms, *J. Bone Jt., Surg.*, 68-B, 36, 1986.

34. **Brinckmann, N. P. and Horst, M.,** The influence of vertebral body fracture, intradiscal injection and partial discectomy on the radial bulge and height of human lumbar discs, *Spine*, 10(2), 138, 1985.

35. **Horst, M. and Brinkmann, P.,** Measurement of the distribution of axial stress on the endplate of the vertebral body, *Spine*, 6, 217, 1981.

36. **Horton, W. G.,** Further observations on the elastic mechanism of the intervertebral disc, *J. Bone Jt. Surg.*, 40-B, 552, 1958.

37. **Roaf, R.,** A study of the mechanics of spinal injuries, *J. Bone Jt. Surg.*, 42-B, 810, 1960.

38. **Nachemson, A. L., Schultz, A. B., and Berkson, H.,** Mechanical properties of human lumbar spine motion segments. Influences of age, sex, disc level and degeneration, *Spine*, 4, 1, 1979.

39. **Brinkmann, P., Frobin, W., Hierholzer, E., and Horst, M.,** Deformation of the vertebral end-plate under axial loading of the spine, *Spine*, 8, 851, 1983.

40. **Nachemson, A.,** In vivo discometry in lumbar discs with irregular nucleograms, *Acta Orthop. Scand.*, 36, 418, 1965.

41. **Perey, O.,** Fracture of the vertebral endplate. A biomedical investigation, *Acta Orthop. Scand.*, Suppl. 25, 1957.

42. **Lin, H. S., Liu, Y. K., and Adams, K. H.,** Mechanical response of the lumbar intervertebral joint under physiological (complex) loading, *J. Bone Jt. Surg.*, 60-A, 41, 1978.

43. **Brown, T., Hansen, R. J., and Yorra, A. J.,** Some mechanical tests on the lumbosacral spine with particular reference to the intervertebral disc, *J. Bone Jt. Surg.*, 39-A, 1135, 1957.

44. **Adams, M. A. and Hutton, W. C.,** The effect of posture on the lumbar spine, *J. Bone Jt. Surg.*, 67-B, 625, 1985.

45. **Pearcy, M. J. and Tibrewal, S. B.,** Lumbar intervertebral disc and ligament deformations measured in vivo, *Clin. Orthop. Relat. Res.*, 191, 281, 1984.

46. **Adams, M. A., and Hutton, W. C.,** Prolapsed intervertebral disc. A hyperflexion injury, *Spine*, 7, 184, 1982.

47. **Adams, M. A. and Hutton, W. C.,** The effect of posture on diffusion into lumbar intervertebral discs, *J. Anat.*, 147, 121, 1986.

48. **Rolander, S. D.,** Motion of the lumbar spine with special reference to the stabilising effect of posterior fusion, *Acta Orthop. Scand.*, Suppl. 90, 1966.

49. **Andersson, G. B. and Schultz, A. B.,** Effects of fluid injection on mechanical properties of intervertebral discs, *J. Biomech.*, 12, 453, 1979.

50. **Spencer, D. L., Miller, J. A. A., and Schultz, A. B.,** The effects of chemonucleolysis on the mechanical properties of the canine lumbar disc, *Spine*, 10, 555, 1985.

51. **Adams, M. A. and Hutton, W. C.,** The mechanical function of the lumbar apophyseal joints, *Spine*, 8, 327, 1983.

52. **Farfan, H. F., Cossette, J. W., Robertson, G. H., Wells, R. V., and Kraus, H.,** The effects of torsion on the lumbar intervertebral joints: the role of torsion in the production of disc degeneration, *J. Bone Jt. Surg.*, 52-A, 468, 1970.

53. **Gregersen, G. G. and Lucas, D. B.,** An in-vivo study of the axial rotation of the human thoracolumbar spine, *J. Bone Jt. Surg.*, 49-A, 247, 1967.

54. **Lumsden, R. M. and Morris, J. M.,** An in-vivo study of axial rotation and immobilisation at the lumbosacral joint, *J. Bone Jt. Surg.*, 50-A, 1591, 1968.

55. **Hardy, W. G., Lissner, H. R., Webster, J. E., and Gurdjian, F. S.,** Repeated loading tests of the lumbar spine: a preliminary report, *Surg. Forum*, 9, 690, 1958.

56. **King, L.-Y., Njus, G., Buckwalter, J., and Wakano, K.,** Fatigue response of lumbar intervertebral joints under axial cyclic loading, *Spine*, 8, 857, 1983.

57. **Jayson, M. I. V., Herbert, C. M., and Barks, J. S.,** Intervertebral discs: nuclear morphology and bursting pressures, *Ann. Rheum. Dis.*, 32, 308, 1973.

58. **Virgin, W. J.,** Experimental investigations into the physical properties of the intervertebral disc, *J. Bone Jt. Surg.*, 33-B, 607, 1951.

59. **Brinkmann, P.,** personal communication, 1985.

60. **Rissanen, P. M.,** The surgical anatomy and pathology of the supraspinous and interspinous ligaments of the lumbar spine with special reference to ligament ruptures, *Acta Orthop. Scand.*, Suppl. 46, 1960.

61. **Adams, M. A. and Hutton, W. C.,** The effects of fatigue on the lumbar intervertebral disc, *J. Bone Jt. Surg.*, 65-B, 199, 1983.

62. **Adams, M. A. and Hutton, W. C.,** Gradual disc prolapse, *Spine*, 10, 524, 1985.

63. **Twomey, L. and Taylor, J.,** Flexion creep deformation and hysteresis in the lumbar vertebral column, *Spine*, 7, 116, 1982.

64. **Bayliss, M. T., Urban, J. P., Johnstone, B., Menage, J., and O'Brien, J. P.,** Proteoglycan synthesis rates in the intervertebral disc, paper presented at the Annu. Meeting Int. Soc. Study of the Lumbar Spine, Sydney, Australia, 1985.
65. **Muir, I. H. M.,** Biochemistry, in *Adult Articular Cartilage,* 2nd ed., Freeman, M. A. R., Ed., Pitman Medical, London, 1979, 145.
66. **Kelsey, J.,** An epidemiological study of acute herniated lumbar intervertebral discs, *Rheumatol. Rehabil.,* 14, 144, 1975.
67. **Troup, J. D. G., Martin, J. W., and Lloyd, D. C. E. F.,** Back pain in industry, *Spine,* 6(1), 61, 1981.
68. **Kelsey, J. L. and White, A. A.,** Epidemiology and impact of low back pain, *Spine,* 5, 133, 1980.
69. **Kraemer, J., Kolditz, D., and Gowin, R.,** Water and electrolyte content of human intervertebral discs under variable load, *Spine,* 10(1), 69, 1985.
70. **Urban, J. P. G.,** Fluid and Solute Transport in the Intervertebral disc, Ph.D. thesis, London University, England, 1977.
71. **Koeller, W., Funke, F., and Hartmann, F.,** Biomechanical behaviour of human intervertebral discs subjected to long-lasting axial loading, *Biorheology,* 21, 675, 1984.
72. **Simon, B. R., Wu, J. S. S., Carlton, M. W., Kazarian, L. E., France, E. P., Evans, J. H., and Zienkiewicz, O. C.,** Poroelastic dynamic structural model of Rhesus spinal motion segments, *Spine,* 10, 495, 1985.
73. **Adams, M. A. and Hutton, W. C.,** The effect of posture on the fluid content of lumbar intervertebral discs, *Spine,* 8, 665, 1983.
74. **Koeller, W., Muehlhaus, S., Meier, W., and Hartman, F.,** personal communication, 1985.
75. **Kazarian, L.,** Creep characteristics of the human spinal column, *Orthop. Clin. N. Am.,* 6, 3, 1975.
76. **Hukins, D. W. L. and Davies, K. E.,** Shape and fibre reinforcing in intervertebral discs related to mechanical function and failure, paper presented at the Ann. Meeting of the Int. Soc. Study Lumbar Spine, Sydney, Australia, 1985.
77. **Koeller, W., Meier, W., and Hartman, F.,** Biomechanical properties of human intervertebral discs subjected to axial dynamic compression. A comparison of lumbar and thoracic discs, *Spine,* 9, 725, 1984.
78. **Tomlinson, N. and Maroudas, A.,** unpublished results, 1983.
79. **Urban, J. P. G., Holm, S., Maroudas, A., and Nachemson, A.,** Nutrition of the intervertebral disc, *Clin. Orthop.,* 129, 101, 1977.
80. **De Pukey, P.,** The physiological oscillation of the length of the body, *Acta Orthop. Scand.,* 6, 338, 1935.
81. **Tyrrell, A. R., Reilly, T., and Troup, J. D. G.,** Circadian variation in stature and the effects of spinal loading, *Spine,* 10, 161, 1985.
82. **Holm, S., Maroudas, A., Urban, J. P. G., Selstam, G., and Nachemson, A.,** Nutrition of the intervertebral disc: effect of fluid flow on solute transport, *Clin. Orthop.,* 170, 296, 1982.
83. **Maroudas, A., Stockwell, R. A., Nachemson, A., and Urban, J.,** Factors involved in the nutrition of the human lumbar intervertebral disc: cellularity and diffusion of glucose in vitro, *J. Anat.,* 120, 113, 1975.
84. **White, A. A. and Panjabi, M. M.,** The basic kinematics of the human spine, *Spine,* 3, 12, 1978.
85. **Pearcy, M., Portek, I., and Shepherd, J.,** Three-dimensional X-ray analysis of normal movement in the lumbar spine, *Spine,* 9, 294, 1984.
86. **Andersson, G. B. J., Murphy, R. W., Ortengren, R., and Nachemson, A. L.,** The influence of backrest inclination and lumbar support on lumbar lordosis, *Spine,* 4, 52, 1979.

Chapter 11

DISC PATHOLOGY AND DISEASE STATES

Barrie Vernon-Roberts

TABLE OF CONTENTS

I. INTRODUCTION

A very large number of congenital, mechanical, inflammatory, degenerative, metabolic, and neoplastic conditions can affect the spine and may be associated with neck or back pain or other symptoms.

Compared with the great frequency of back pain in the population, opportunities for the pathological examination of the discs occur on very infrequent occasions during life. Moreover, there are still relatively few publications dealing with the pathological features of the spine post-mortem even with respect to the condition which is universally present in the adult population, namely, lumbar spondylosis. The past 2 decades, however, have seen a burgeoning interest in back pain and its causation, and this has been accompanied by an increasing number of scientific meetings and a rapidly increasing literature devoted to the spine. Despite this widespread awakening to the prevalence and social and economic importance of back pain, and the clinical application of many new diagnostic and treatment procedures, a mere trickle of new information has come forth defining the pathological changes in the component parts of the spine. The relative paucity of pathological information testifies to the many difficulties faced in attempting to obtain spinal tissues suitable for comprehensive pathological examination and the problems of attempting to correlate post-mortem anatomic pathology of the spine with back pain symptoms occurring during life.

These difficulties notwithstanding, it is clear from published accounts available hitherto that the intervertebral discs exhibit a wide range of macroscopic and microscopic features which, in some instances, can be correlated with specific diseases or syndromes. The major problem in determining the clinical significance of pathological features in the discs, however, continues to be the universal presence of spondylosis encountered in the adult population at autopsy, and the high frequency with which vertical and posterior disc protrusions are found during detailed examination of post-mortem material. Because of this overlap, problems exist for the pathologist in attempting to ascribe features encountered to specific disease states, and due caution must be exercised in this regard. Nevertheless, as new imaging techniques are refined, it is likely that, in the near future, it will become increasingly possible to correlate clinical symptomatology with specific structural changes identified by organ imaging, and to account for the latter by demonstrable pathological changes in the discs.

Against this background, this chapter sets out to provide accounts of structural changes in the discs known to occur in various disease states. It must be borne in mind, moreover, that the discs are only one component of a complex anatomical structure and it is rarely the case that the discs are the only vertebral components which undergo changes, and that pathological changes in the discs may occur only rarely in some diseases which predominantly affect other body systems. For the purpose of completeness, it will be necessary to succinctly state the clinical features of each condition. For obvious reasons, the attention devoted to each condition will reflect its prevalence and the body of knowledge concerning structural changes in the discs.

II. SPONDYLOSIS

A. Clinical

The term "spondylosis" (synonyms: degenerative spondylosis, spondylosis deformans, spinal osteophytosis) is applied to a spectrum of changes affecting one or multiple levels signified radiologically by narrowing of the disc (loss of disc height), osteophytes arising from the margins of the vertebral bodies, and osteoarthritic changes in the apophyseal (posterior intervertebral and zygapophyseal) joints. The condition may be primary, usually affecting several levels of the lumbar or, less commonly, the cervical spine, or may be secondary to structural abnormalities or to previous trauma or inflammation. Spondylosis frequently is asymptomatic but sometimes may be associated with various pain syndromes which are usually nonspecific; however, symptoms indicating nerve root compression or spinal stenosis may be present.

B. Incidence

Autopsy studies report considerably higher percentages of the incidence of spondylosis than do clinical radiological studies. The largely macroscopic examination of 4253 spines obtained at autopsy by Schmorl revealed evidence of the condition in 60% of females and 80% of males by the age of 49 years and in 95% of both sexes by the age of 70 years. Other studies indicate that, compared with young normal discs, microscopic, and occasionally macroscopic, evidence of significant structural damage is present in the lumbar discs by the 3rd decade in the large majority of, if not all, spines.[1-10]

The differences in the frequency of spondylosis in clinical radiological studies compared with pathological studies are due to the inability of routine radiographic techniques to demonstrate the presence of small bony spurs and to the need for disc changes to be relatively advanced before they are revealed by discography. While CT scanning, ultrasound, and stereoscopic radiography are capable of visualizing more discrete changes in spinal components, the recently developed technique of nuclear magnetic resonance imaging offers the possibility of soon being able to detect early biochemical and structural changes in the component parts of the discs.

C. Spondylosis: Age-Related Degeneration or Pathological Process?

Since greater or lesser degrees of structural changes in the discs are universal by middle life, semantic questions directed toward ascertaining whether spondylosis should be regarded as a degenerative (or inevitable age-related process) or a pathological sequence following some potentially identifiable initiating stimulus or stimuli are often posed. While there is evidence that acquired structural abnormalities of the disc occurring early in life, such as vertical or posterior protrusions, may be associated with the earlier onset of advanced spondylosis, the initiating events remain obscure despite some biochemical studies. There is, however, wide agreement that the initial changes of spondylosis occur within the disc, closely followed by osteophyte formation on the rims of the vertebral bodies and osteoarthritic changes in the apophyseal joints at the level of the affected disc.

D. Structure of the Young Normal (Predegenerate) Disc

Consideration of the structural changes in the disc in spondylosis is facilitated by an understanding of the macroscopic and microscopic anatomy of the young (predegenerate) disc with respect to its major components: the nucleus, the annulus fibrosus, and the end-plates.

In childhood, the opposing vertebral bodies are completely covered by thin plates of cartilage forming the epiphysis. After puberty, secondary centers of ossification appear in these epiphyses and fuse with the primary bone after the age of 21 years. However, they ossify only the periphery (the marginal ring) of the cartilaginous plates, the central part remaining cartilaginous. In advanced life, this central portion may become partly or wholly ossified. Thus, in the adult, the bony end-plates of the opposing vertebral bodies usually are covered centrally by thin laminae of hyaline cartilage known as the hyaline laminae or cartilage end-plates. The cartilage end-plates, up to 1 mm in thickness, abut onto the nucleus pulposus, while the surrounding rim of bone, up to 1 cm in width, forms the major site of attachment of the annulus fibrosus to the bone.

The annulus fibrosus is largely composed of discrete concentric layers of fibrous tissue inserted into the bone of the vertebral rim (the marginal ring) in a strong attachment known as an enthesis. The fibers of each layer are parallel and run spirally at an angle of 45° to

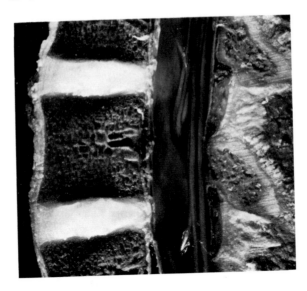

FIGURE 1. Portion of bisected lumbar spine from 25-year-old individual. Compared with young discs, the clear distinction between the nucleus and annulus of each disc no longer exists, and the nuclei no longer bulge from the cut surface of the discs.

the bodies of the vertebrae, and the fibers of alternate layers are at right angles to each other.[10] This arrangement results in great strength of union of the vertebral bodies, while, at the same time, the criss-cross arrangement of fibers resists torsional and flexional deformity and ensures resistance to rupture of the annulus. The annulus is thin at birth, but extends centripetally during life. Sparse blood vessels and nerves normally extend between the layers of the outer third of the annulus, but the inner two thirds normally lack a blood and nerve supply. The posterior longitudinal ligament, which runs down the posterior surfaces of the vertebral bodies inside the spinal canal, is firmly united to the posterior surface of the annulus by lateral expansion of the ligament. The anterior longitudinal ligament, which runs down the front of the spine, is not attached to the anterior annulus.

Enclosed by the annulus is the nucleus pulposus, the shape of which in the horizontal plane is determined by the annulus being thickest anteriorly and thinnest posterolaterally resulting in the nucleus being kidney-shaped. The normal young adult disc does not contain blood vessels or nerves, and the disc is largely nourished by diffusion from vessels located under the bony end-plates adjoining the hyaline laminae.[11] In older individuals, it is not unusual to find small vessels crossing the bony end-plate and extending into or through the cartilage end-plate.

At birth, the discs consist almost entirely of nucleus with a thin surrounding annulus. In childhood and adolescence, the nuclei are gelatinous and turgid so that the contents bulge spontaneously from the freshly cut surface at autopsy. In childhood, the nuclei are composed predominantly of semigelatinous material traversed by few delicate collagen fibers and sometimes contain stellate chordal cells in addition to the dominant population of cells morphologically similar to chondrocytes and some fibroblast-type cells. By the third decade, the nuclei are semisolid and have lost much of their turgescence (Figures 1 and 2). Microscopy shows that this is associated with the centripetal encroachment of collagen in continuity with the inner region of the annulus and a reduction in the number of cells in the nucleus. After middle life, in the majority of spines examined, the nuclei are solid, nonturgescent, dry, and granular to the touch; they are often brown in color, and have merged with the annulus so that a clear distinction between the nucleus and annulus is not possible. Further loss of

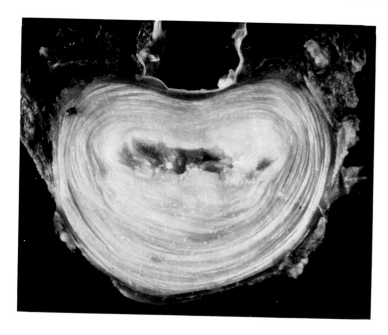

FIGURE 2. Surface of horizontally divided lumbar disc in 25-year-old individual showing the concentric bands of annular fibers which have encroached centripetally upon the nucleus. Only a small portion of the nucleus remains gelatinous.

nuclear cells takes place during the development of these later changes. While many consider that the disc loses vertical height during adult life, recent studies have challenged this assumption.

E. Age-Related Degenerative Changes

Compared with the appearance of the normal disc prior to the third decade, a spectrum of structural abnormalities may be seen macroscopically and microscopically in all the component parts of the disc in older individuals as the age-related condition of spondylosis develops and progresses. However, it should be borne in mind that spondylosis may develop at an earlier age or progress more rapidly when other structural abnormalities are present, that the onset of significant structural changes may take place at different ages in different individuals, and that the progression or extent of involvement differs widely from individual to individual. In general, the changes are most marked in the lumbar spine, appearing earlier and progressing more rapidly in the lowest disc, and are more marked in the cervical than the thoracic spine.

In the nucleus pulposus, the earliest macroscopic change appears to be the appearance of splits and clefts about midway between the center of the disc and the cartilage end-plates, and generally oriented parallel to the end-plates (Figure 3). The upper and lower clefts tend to extend posteriorly, where they may merge, and posterolaterally, where they are associated with disruption and thinning of the annulus fibrosus (Figure 4). Thus, as the clefts enlarge, they may isolate progressively the central portion of the disc from the surrounding disc tissue; occasionally, the merging of upper and lower clefts can lead to a portion of the central disc becoming isolated to form a loose body contained within a cavitated portion of the disc. The posterior and posterolateral extension of the clefts frequently pass through the annular fibers (Figures 4 and 5) and may extend to the peridural space of the spinal canal (Figure 6). They also frequently extend to the bony attachment of the annular fibers anteriorly or posteriorly (or both), where they may be associated with a cleft in the bony end-plate

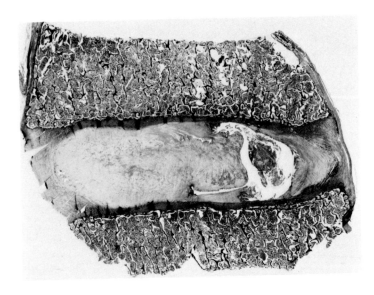

FIGURE 3. Very low-power microscopic view of sagittal section of lumbar disc and adjacent vertebral bodies. Degeneration has occurred in the posterior region of the disc (right), and clefts have extended anteriorly in parallel with the end-plates above and below.

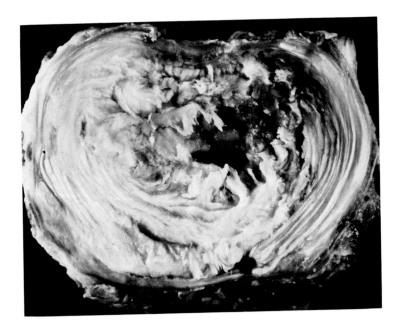

FIGURE 4. Surface of horizontally divided lumbar disc in 40-year-old individual. Shows a central defect in the nucleus due to cleft formation and irregular fissures passing into the surrounding nucleus and annulus. A circumferential cleft is present in the middle zone of the anterior (bottom of photograph) region of the annulus.

(Figure 6) and chronic inflammatory reaction in the adjacent marrow tissue (Figure 7). Those clefts which transgress the annulus rarely contain nuclear material and are unlikely, therefore, to have been formed by a process of nuclear herniation.

The enlargement of clefts and their extension to involve the annulus produces cavities and cystic spaces of varying size and shape within the disc (Figures 4, 8, and 9).

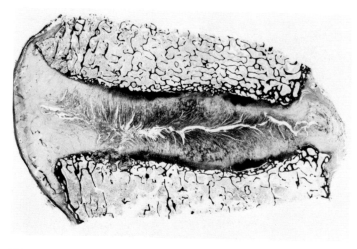

FIGURE 5. Very low-power microscopic view of section of lumbar disc and adjacent vertebral bodies. There is an extensive central cleft passing horizontally and extending nearly through the posterior annulus (right) and deeply into the anterior annulus (left).

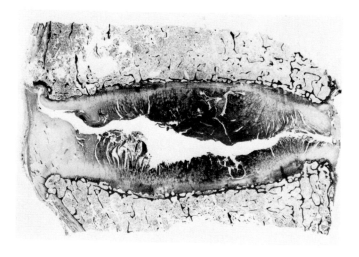

FIGURE 6. Very low-power microscopic view of section of lumbar disc and adjacent vertebral bodies. There is a large central cleft passing through the posterior annulus (right). The cleft also passes deeply through the anterior annulus (left) and has extended through the outer annular attachment into the rim of the upper vertebral body. Note the frond-like fissuring of areas of the nucleus at the margins of the cleft.

Microscopic examination of the nucleus suggests that the clefts usually begin in the region of the posterior zone of the nucleus near its junction with the annulus, and that their appearance is associated with degenerative changes in the nucleus indicated by loss of metachromasia and death of chondrocytes. When the clefts have become established, the margins of the clefts frequently are formed of fissured nuclear material with clusters of proliferated chondrocytes (chondrones; Figures 6 and 10); these appearances are very similar to those of osteoarthritic articular cartilage in the stage of advanced fibrillation. Rarely, the clefts may have acquired a lining layer similar in appearance to the lining of synovial membrane. When clefts pass deeply into the annulus, microscopy occasionally reveals the ingrowth of blood vessels, accompanied by nerves, around the margins of a cleft (Figure

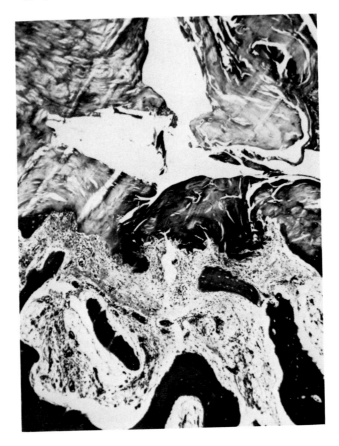

FIGURE 7.   Higher magnification of Figure 6 showing the area where the cleft extends through the anterior annulus to the bone of the vertebral rim. Note the disorganization of the annular attachment, the disappearance of part of the bony end-plate, and the inflammatory reaction in the adjoining marrow tissues.

11). Thus, the normally avascular and aneural disc may acquire a blood and nerve supply by ingrowth from the outer annular region following cleft formation. The vascular ingrowth rarely may be associated with calcification or ossification within the nucleus.

In the annulus fibrosus, macroscopic changes are not readily discernible (Figure 2) until nuclear changes are advanced, but changes occur early at a microscopic level. Among the microscopic changes which may be observed are fragmentation of fibers (Figure 12), mucinous degeneration of the fibers (Figure 13) leading to cyst formation (Figures 14 and 15), the development of concentric cracks and cavities (which may appear as early as the second decade), and focal aggregation of the collagen to form rounded aggregates of hyaline-like amorphous material (Figure 16).

Almost certainly more important mechanically than these microscopic features are various types of tears involving the annulus. Annular tears occurring at the corners of the vertebral bodies at right angles to the annular fibers (Figures 17, 18, and 19), thus separating the annulus from the marginal rim of the vertebral body, have been described by some authors[9,12,13] and are termed vertebral rim lesions. They are rare in subjects under the age of 30 years, but thereafter the frequency increases with age so that they are commonly present after the age of 50 years. They are considered to arise from focal traumatic avulsion of the annulus, possibly secondary to focal degenerative weakening of the annulus; and larger rim lesions

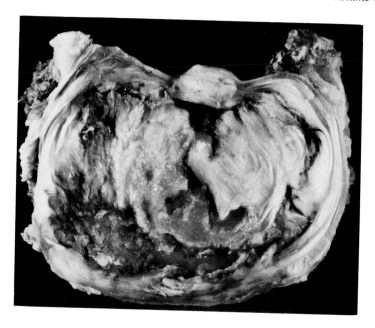

FIGURE 8.   Surface of horizontally divided lumbar disc showing advanced changes with large, irregular defects present in the nucleus and extensively involving the anterior annulus (lower part of photograph).

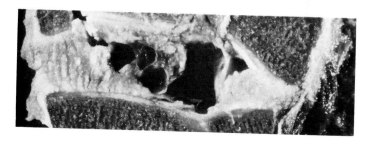

FIGURE 9.   Photograph of bisected lumbar disc showing extensive cystic cavitation of the central region of the disc in an elderly individual.

may be recognized radiographically by the presence of the vacuum phenomenon, vertebral rim sclerosis with or without a cup-shaped defect in the rim, and osteophytes confined to one side of the disc.[13] Rim lesions may be accompanied by ingrowth of vascular and granulation tissue into the annulus (Figure 20) and replacement of portions of the bony attachment of the annulus by granulation tissue (Figures 21, 22).

The rim lesions differ from the commonly present concentric cracks and cavities, which, in turn, differ from the macroscopically visible annular ruptures extending radially from the nucleus toward the periphery (Figures 23 and 24), which are known as "radiating ruptures".[5,6] Radiating ruptures are frequently present between the ages of 30 and 50 years and most frequently involve the posterior zones of the lower lumbar discs. When these ruptures transgress the annulus, there frequently follows the ingrowth of vascular tissue (Figure 25) along the site of the rupture. According to some reports,[6] this vascularization process may lead to healing with scar tissue formation if the rupture is small, but does not lead to healing if the rupture is extensive (Figure 26). It would appear from the age of incidence, frequency, morphology, and localization that radiating ruptures of the annulus and cleft formation in

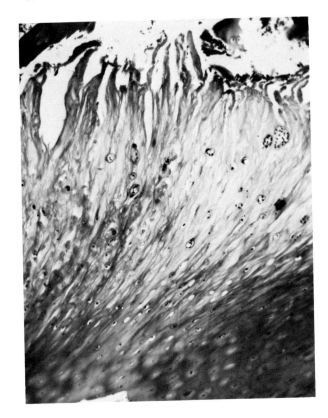

FIGURE 10.   Medium-power microscopic view of margin of a cleft.
The cavity formed by the cleft is shown in the upper part of the field,
and the disc substance bordering on the cleft shows marked fissuring and
contains clusters of proliferated chondrocytes. These appearances are
similar to those in articular cartilage in advanced osteoarthritis.

the nucleus should not, in most instances, be regarded as separate processes, but probably
are interrelated phenomena consequent upon solidification and cracking of the disc combined
with degeneration and repeated trauma sustained by the annulus.

In addition to the commonly present Schmorl's nodes (considered later in this chapter)
the end-plate region also exhibits a spectrum of changes which become more frequent and
marked during the 3rd decade.[2] Early changes in the cartilage end-plate are fissure formation,
fractures (Figure 27), horizontal cleft formation which is sometimes extensive (Figure 28),
death of chondrocytes, increased vascular penetration (Figure 29), and extension of calcification and ossification from the bony end-plate (Figure 30). Later, there is progressive
loss of the cartilage with vascularization and ossification, and microscopic protrusions of
nuclear material through defects in the cartilage (without breaching of the bony end-plate;
Figure 31). During and after the 5th decade, frequently there has been extensive or total
loss of the cartilage end-plate, many clefts and fissures are present in the residual cartilage,
protrusions of nuclear material are common, and islands of new cartilage are encountered
on the vertebral side of the bony end-plate (Figure 32). Irregular ossification results in
variations in the thickness and profile of the underlying bony end-plates, and double bony
end-plates may develop.[9]

F. Vertebral Body Osteophytes

As the discs degenerate, osteophytic outgrowths of varying size inevitably form on the
anterior and anterolateral margins of the vertebral bodies and may become very large as

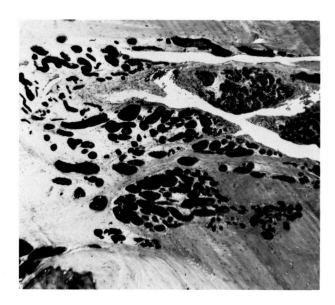

FIGURE 11. Low-power microscopic view of clefts extending into the anterior annulus. There are numerous blood vessels (appearing black in the micrograph) growing into the disc along the margins of the clefts.

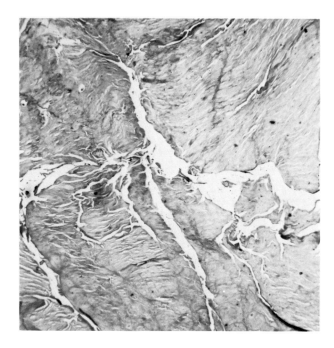

FIGURE 12. Low-power microscopic view of annulus showing a focus of fragmentation of the annular fibers.

"beaked" or "kissing" osteophytes. The stimulus to their formation remains speculative. Collins[14] proposed that such osteophytes formed as a result of elevation of periosteum caused by a forward squeezing out of disc substance by tilting of the vertebral bodies owing to the narrowing of the disc through degeneration. Microscopic studies, however, do not provide support for the concept of subperiosteal new bone formation and indicate that the marginal

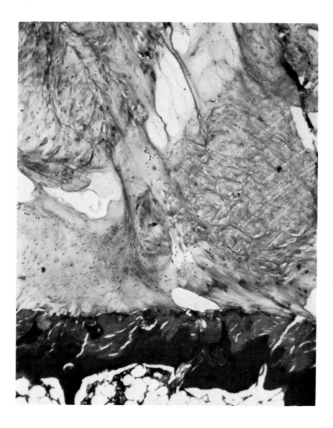

FIGURE 13.   Low-power microscopic view of region of attachment of annulus (upper part of field) to the bone of the vertebral body (lower part of field). Extensive mucinous degeneration of the annular fibers has led to the formation of cystic spaces.

osteophytes form, at least initially, by the endochondral ossification of metaplastic cartilage appearing within the annulus in the region of the anterior attachments of the annulus to the bone (Figure 33).[9]

When disc degeneration is advanced and a significant degree of disc thinning has occurred, large osteophytic flanges may involve the lateral and posterior region also, may compromise the nerve roots emerging from the spinal canal, and may contribute to the development of lateral nerve entrapment and spinal stenosis syndromes (Figure 35).[10,15] However, unlike the commonly occurring bony ankylosis of syndesmophytes in ankylosing spondylosis *(vide infra),* it is very rarely the case that even very large osteophytes undergo bony fusion, although they may effectively impede movements between the vertebral bodies.

G. Disc Thinning

While views have been expressed recently that disc thinning (loss of disc height) is not normally a feature of spondylosis, this would not have wide acceptance from pathologists or radiologists. It probably results from the examination of some older spines in which advanced osteoporotic changes present in the vertebral bodies (''codfish'' vertebrae) are associated with a ballooning of the discs. In advanced osteoporosis, it is not uncommonly the case that minimal spondylitic changes are present at an advanced age, and this has allowed speculation as to the protective effect of the reduced bone stiffness in preventing or delaying disc degeneration.

In advanced spondylosis, the discs frequently are thinned. Many factors may contribute

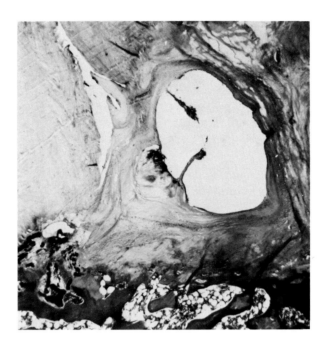

FIGURE 14. Low-power microscopic view of region of annular attachment to the vertebral body. A large cystic space has formed within the annulus.

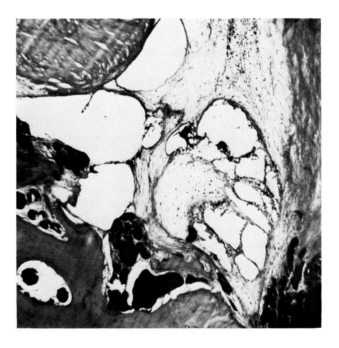

FIGURE 15. Low-power microscopic view of region of annular attachment to the vertebral body. Numerous cystic spaces have formed within the annulus and blood vessels have extended into the tissues surrounding the cysts.

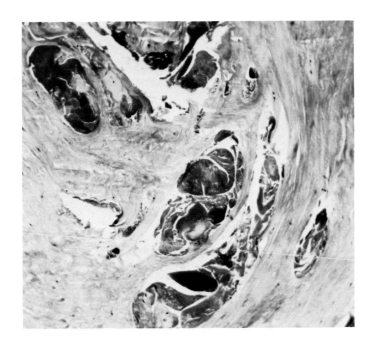

FIGURE 16.   Low-power microscopic view of outer region of anterior annulus showing extensive focal aggregation of the collagen to form masses of amorphous degenerate material.

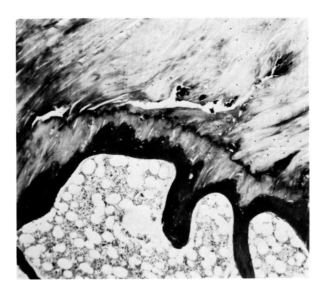

FIGURE 17.   Low-power microscopic view of region of annular attachment to the vertebral body. There is a transverse tear of the annulus at the site of the attachment of the annular fibers to the underlying rim of the vertebral body.

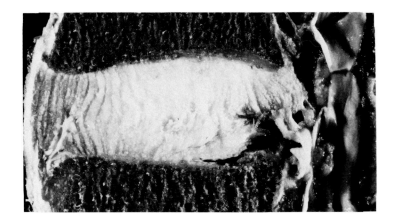

FIGURE 18. Photograph of bisected lumbar disc showing a large vertebral rim lesion formed as a result of tearing of the posterior annular fibers at their attachment to the inferior vertebral rim.

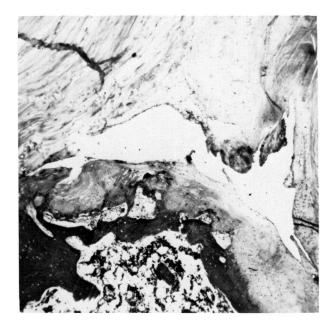

FIGURE 19. Low-power microscopic view of region of annular attachment to the vertebral body showing an extensive defect at the site of the attachment of the annular fibers to the vertebral rim.

to this, including a reduction in water content, the progressive conversion of the nucleus to a highly collagenized tissue as age advances, protrusion of disc tissue, ossification of the cartilage end–plate, and, possibly, the partial replacement of the disc by vascular granulation tissue eventually maturing to form fibrous scar-type tissue occupying a smaller volume than the original disc substance. These processes, commonly resulting in disc thinning in advanced spondylosis (Figure 34), probably should be distinguished from the condition which has been described as isolated disc resorption,[16] which tends to be restricted to the L5—S1 disc and meets certain radiological criteria.[17]

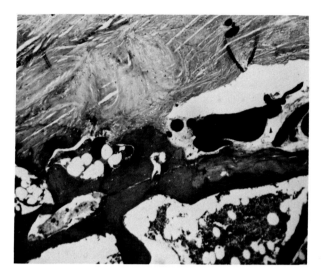

FIGURE 20.   Low-power microscopic view of region of annular attachment to the vertebral body. Shows blood vessels (appearing black in the micrograph) which have extended along the margin of an annular tear.

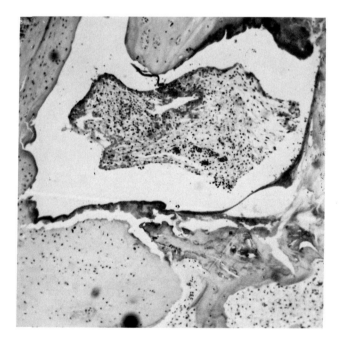

FIGURE 21.   Low-power microscopic view of region of annular attachment to the vertebral body. Shows a large cavity in the annulus largely occupied by granulation tissue.

H. Apophyseal Joints and Lateral and Central Stenosis

While a detailed description of the apophyseal joints in spondylosis lies outside the terms of reference of the chapter, it needs to be stressed that the spinal segments displaying the advanced degenerative changes in the discs described above always show osteoarthritic changes to some degree in the apophyseal joints at the same level.[9,10,15,18] These changes

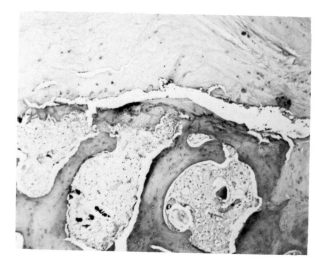

FIGURE 22. Low-power microscopic view of region of annular attachment to the vertebral body. There is an extensive tear separating the annulus from the bone. The marrow spaces in the adjoining bone are occupied by granulation tissue which is also replacing areas of the bony end-plate.

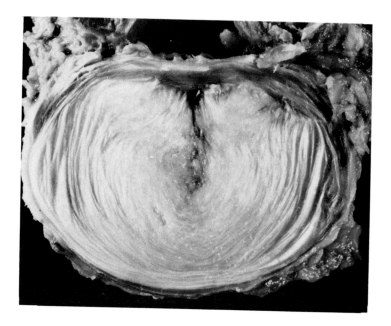

FIGURE 23. Surface of horizontally divided lumbar disc in 35-year-old individual. There is an annular rupture extending from the center of the disc toward the midline posteriorly.

have led to the concept of the two posterior joints and the disc as a functionally and pathologically interrelated three-joint complex existing at each level.[15] It is important that the combination of changes in the disc and posterior joints sometimes produces entrapment of a spinal nerve in the lateral recess, central stenosis at one level, or both of these conditions (Figure 35).[15] Changes at one level usually lead, over a period of years, to multilevel spondylosis and stenosis.

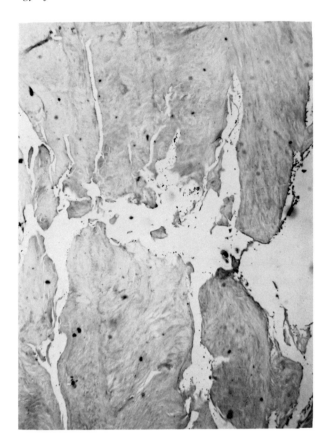

FIGURE 24. Low-power microscopic view of portion of posterior annulus showing an irregular tear separating the ruptured annular fibers.

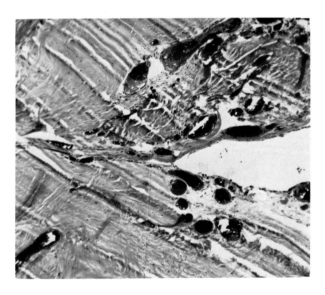

FIGURE 25. Low-power microscopic view showing blood vessels (appearing black in the micrograph) extending along the margins of an annular rupture.

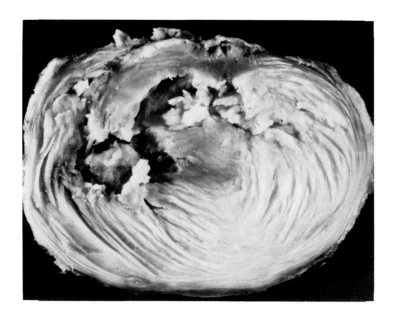

FIGURE 26.   Surface of horizontally divided lumbar disc in 50-year-old individual showing an extensive rupture of the lateral portion of annulus.

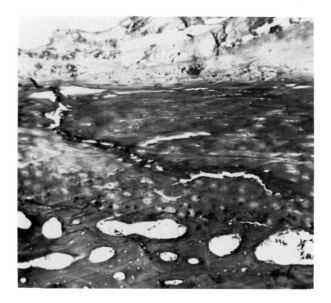

FIGURE 27.   Low-power microscopic view of the central end-plate zone. There is an oblique fracture extending diagonally through the hyaline lamina between the degenerated nucleus (above) and the bony end-plate (below).

III. DISC PROTRUSION: PROLAPSE AND HERNIATION

A. Clinical

It is clear that there is a constant tendency to displacement of the nucleus due to the forces acting on it. Normally the cartilage end-plates and the annulus are sufficiently strong to prevent displacement of the nucleus even under conditions of great stress. In all discs,

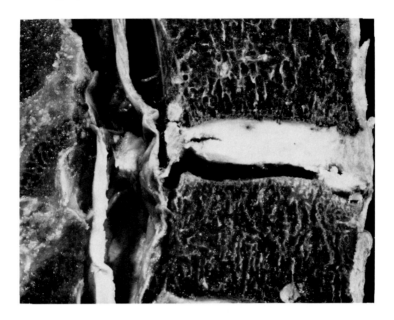

FIGURE 28. Photograph of disc in bisected lumbar spine showing extensive separation of the disc from the vertebral body above by a very large horizontal cleft.

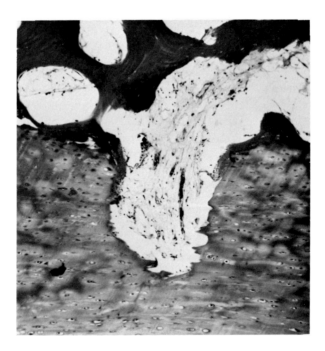

FIGURE 29. Medium-power microscopic view of portion of central end-plate zone. Vascular tissue has extended from the bony end-plate (above) into the cartilage end-plate toward the nucleus (below).

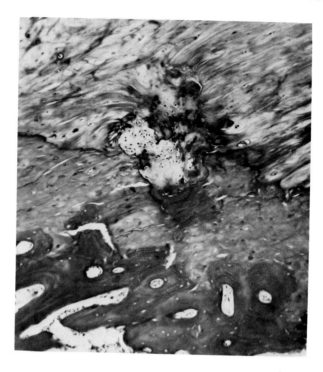

FIGURE 30.   Medium-power microscopic view of portion of central end-plate zone. Ossification is taking place in the cartilage end-plate as vessels extend into the disc (above) from the bony end-plate region (below).

however, there are two potentially weak points: (1) the cartilage end-plate, which is supported by the very thin subchondral bone plate and the underlying trabecular bone; and (2) the posterior and posterolateral segments of the annulus, which not only are thinner than the anterior and lateral segments but also are less firmly attached to the bone. It is at these two points that herniation is liable to occur.

Lateral or anterior ruptures of the annulus are probably rare. By contrast, anterolateral bulging (without rupture) of the annulus is a frequent occurrence after extrusion of the nucleus in another direction (posteriorly or vertically) has caused the disc to collapse; it occurs anteriorly because of the forward tilting of the vertebral bodies pivoting on the apophyseal joints and laterally because of the presence in the midline of the anterior longitudinal ligament.[14]

It seems likely that herniation is associated with an episode of trauma. It may be that congenital or acquired defects of the cartilage end-plates or posterior annulus are predisposing factors in some cases. It is clear that herniation of the nucleus is more likely to occur when it is still turgescent and is less likely after middle age, when the nucleus has become desiccated and collagenized.

While vertical disc protrusions (Schmorl's nodes) are very commonly encountered during pathological studies of the spine *(vide infra)*, it is not clear whether the evolution of a Schmorl's node gives rise to pain or other symptoms. Schmorl's nodes have been noted to be present in adolescent kyphosis (Scheuermann's disease and vertebral epiphysitis)[12] and spondyloepiphyseal dysplasia,[19] but their frequency in the normal population is so high as to throw doubt on a possible specific etiopathological role in either of these conditions. However, disc degeneration occurs at an earlier age and is more frequent in discs with Schmorl's nodes,[20] and thus Schmorl's nodes contribute to the earlier development of spondylosis.

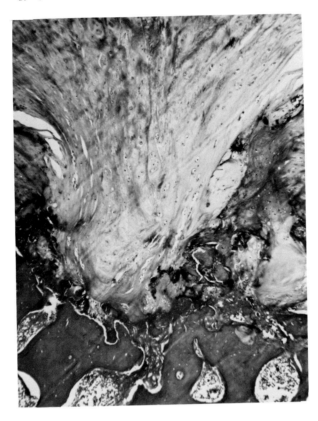

FIGURE 31.   Medium-power photograph of central end-plate zone showing vertical protrusion of nuclear material through the cartilage end-plate. The protrusion has not passed through the bony end-plate (lower part of the field).

Because they may impinge on nerve roots or pain-sensitive structures, posterior protrusions (prolapsed intervertebral discs) are often associated with symptoms despite occurring less frequently than vertical protrusions. Posterior protrusions of cervical discs usually occur in young people and are associated with the acute onset of severe pain in the neck and shoulder accompanied by asymmetric reduction of movement and marked muscular spasm (acute torticollis). The lower discs, commonly C7, tend to be affected, and a neurological deficit may be evident. The condition usually resolves spontaneously within a few days, and conservative treatment only is required in most instances. Acute posterior protrusions of lumbar discs usually affect young adults (aged 20 to 50 years) and frequently give rise to pain (lumbago) due to impingement on the spinal dura mater or nerve root sheath with pain and paresthesiae distributed down the leg (sciatica). In most patients, the lumbago settles spontaneously in a few days, but operative intervention may be required to remove the pressure on the neural tissues.

Anterior protrusions are rare and are not known to be associated with identifiable symptoms.

B. Vertical Protrusions: Schmorl's Nodes

Schmorl's nodes[21,22] are frequently found at autopsy when the vertebral bodies are bisected (Figure 36). Schmorl himself found them in about 38% of all spines examined.[12] Men were involved more frequently (39.9%) than women (34.3%). Between the ages of 18 and 59 years they were twice as common in men as in women, but after the age of 60 they were twice as common in women as in men.

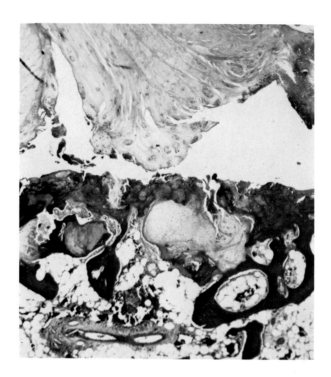

FIGURE 32.   Low-power microscopic view of an end-plate zone showing a large irregular horizontal cleft separating the disc (above) from the
bony end-plate (below). Islands of new cartilage are present on the
vertebral side of the end-plate.

Coventry et al.[23] reported a higher overall incidence, 64%, in a study of 88 spines and
stated that while no spines examined in the 1st decade showed Schmorl's nodes, they were
present in 25 spines in the 3rd decade, 55% in the 4th decade, and about 75% of the 5th
decade and thereafter. However, more recent autopsy studies have reported that not only
are Schmorl's nodes present in 76% of spines, but they are present with equal frequency in
subjects above and below the age of 50 years.[20] The recent findings are consistent with the
view that the majority of Schmorl's nodes are probably present from an early age and only
a small percentage forms in adult life. This supports the concept that herniation of nuclear
material is more likely to occur at an age when the nucleus is in a semifluid state. Discs
having Schmorl's nodes tend to exhibit advanced degenerative changes at an early age, and,
in some instances, at least, the earliest degenerative changes are in the region of the herniation
(Figures 37, 38, and 39).[9]

In marked contrast to the frequency of Schmorl's nodes demonstrable at autopsy, Schmorl's
nodes are demonstrable by clinical radiography in only about 13.5% of cases.[12] The majority
of Schmorl's nodes cannot be detected in clinical radiographs because the herniations are
too small to produce visible changes, or the loss of tissue from the nucleus is not large
enough to produce appreciable narrowing of the intervertebral (disc) space. The demon-
stration of Schmorl's nodes radiographically may only be possible when the prolapse is large
enough to produce visible loss of vertebral body bone, and tomography may be necessary
to establish the true nature of the lesion. In fact, Schmorl's nodes are more easily diagnosed
radiographically when they become surrounded, first by a reactive cartilaginous casing, and
later by an osseous casing. Moreover, in a proportion of cases, prolapse is eventually followed
by vascularization (Figure 40), fibrosis, calcification, and ossification of the extruded nuclear
material, and this process may extend into the disc itself (Figures 41 and 42).

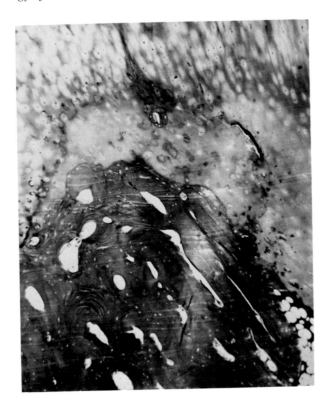

FIGURE 33.   Medium-power microscopic view of osteophyte forming on the vertebral rim. The bone of the osteophyte (the lower half of the field) is being formed by ossification of new cartilage forming at the site of the annular attachment.

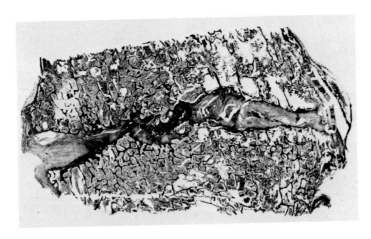

FIGURE 34.   Very low-power microscopic view of section of lumbar disc and adjacent vertebral bodies showing irregular thinning of disc due to marked loss of disc material.

The protrusion of nuclear material cranially or caudally into the adjacent vertebral body is only possible when there is a gap in the cartilage end-plate and subchondral bone plate. Normal (young) cartilage end-plates do not have gaps. Congenital weaknesses of the cartilage end-plates may predispose to gap formation; thus, in some instances, the cartilage opposite the nucleus is much thinner than normal, or a fibrous scar may be present where the end-

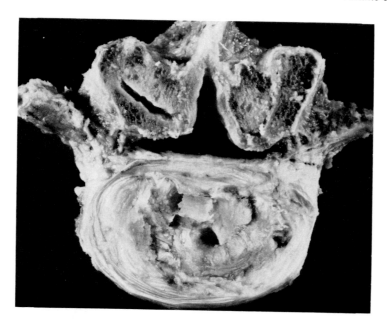

FIGURE 35. Surface of horizontally divided lower lumbar spine in advanced spondylosis. The disc shows marked degeneration, and the posterior intervertebral joints show the changes of advanced osteoarthritis. The spinal canal has become trefoil-shaped due to the combination of changes in the disc and intervertebral joints, and there is a marked elongation of the lateral recesses.

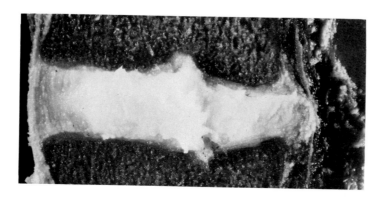

FIGURE 36. Photograph of bisected lumbar disc in an adolescent showing vertical protrusions of nuclear material (Schmorl's nodes) into the vertebral bodies above and below. The disc does not show any macroscopic degenerative features.

plate was perforated by the axial vessels of the disc in embryonic life. However, apart from those rare conditions in young persons associated with the presence of multiple nodes (adolescent kyphosis and Scheuermann's disease), it seems likely that the majority of Schmorl's nodes are the result of acquired lesions of the cartilage end-plate. While microscopic extrusions of nuclear material through the cartilage end-plate may occur in relation to the age-related degeneration and fissuring described previously, it is probable that most herniations occur as a direct result of single or repeated episodes of trauma causing the extrusion of nuclear tissue through tears in the cartilage of the end-plate and fractures in the subjacent subchondral bone. While the usual stresses of everyday life[24] may be sufficient to induce a

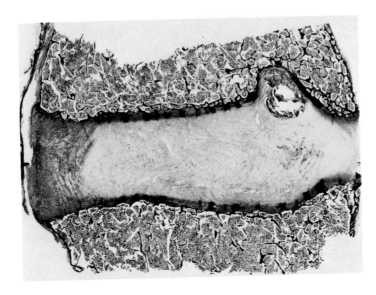

FIGURE 37. Very low-power microscopic view of section of lumbar disc and adjacent vertebral bodies. There is a Schmorl's node formed by herniation of the nucleus into the vertebral body above in the posterior region of the disc. The herniated portion of the disc shows degenerative changes, while the rest of the disc appears normal.

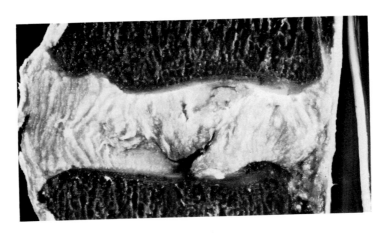

FIGURE 38. Photograph of bisected lumbar disc showing cleft formation commencing in the region of a Schmorl's node present in the central region of the disc.

tear in a previously damaged or abnormal end-plate, there is also no doubt that a single severe traumatic episode may be sufficient to rupture a previously normal healthy disc. In those few cases where it has been possible to carry out a pathological examination of a recently injured spine (Figure 43), it is occasionally possible to find tears in the cartilage end-plates associated with herniation of nuclear tissue into the adjoining bone, causing fractures of trabeculae and surrounding hemorrhage.

Schmorl's nodes rarely are more than 5 mm in diameter, and the majority are much smaller. Most are balloon- or mushroom-shaped since the nuclear material spreads out after passing through a relatively small defect in the cartilage end-plate. They are usually situated slightly posterior to the central axis of the vertebral body, although small nodes are not

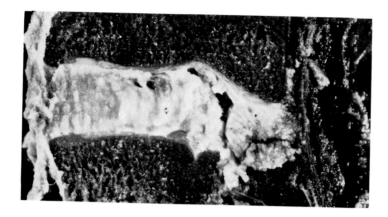

FIGURE 39. Photograph of bisected lumbar disc showing extensive cleft formation in association with the presence of Schmorl's nodes. An extension of the inferior cleft passes through the posterior annulus (right).

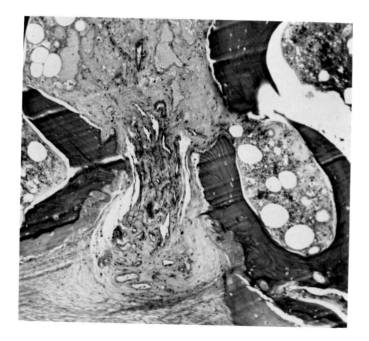

FIGURE 40. Low-power microscopic view of Schmorl's node showing new blood vessels extending from vascularized herniated material present in the vertebral body (above) through the defect in the end-plate into the disc (below).

infrequently seen in other positions. After the extrusion of nuclear material, it is generally considered that the following pathological changes occur. At first, a cavity containing the extruded material is created by fracture of trabeculae and necrosis of marrow tissues in the immediate area of the prolapse. An inflammatory reaction is set up around the herniated material, and there is resorption of necrotic bone and marrow. The enlargement of the prolapse may continue rapidly or slowly in this way until the forces causing further herniation disappear or are successfully opposed by reactive changes surrounding the prolapse. Thus, the further progression and pressure changes that cause enlargement of the disc prolapse are arrested as soon as the nucleus loses its turgescence as a result of age changes, a decrease

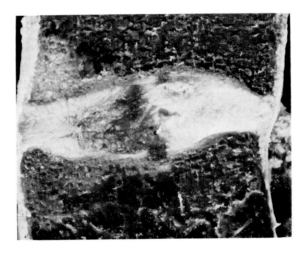

FIGURE 41.   Photograph of bisected lumbar disc showing an extensive dark area of vascularization of the central region of the disc by vessels extending from a Schmorl's node present in the center of the lower end-plate.

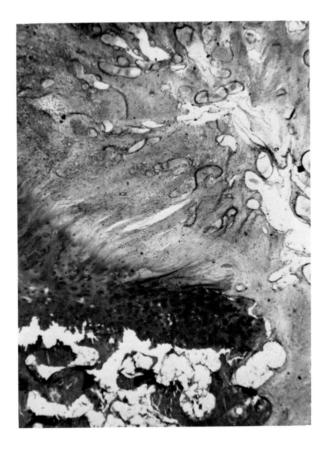

FIGURE 42.   Low-power microscopic view showing extensive blood vessels present within the nucleus (above). These vessels have gained access to the disc (below) through the defect in the end-plate.

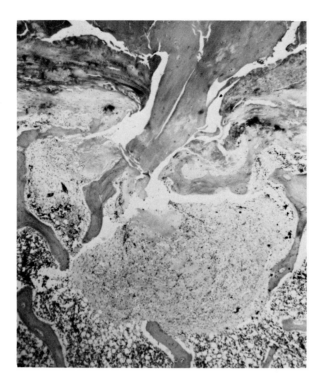

FIGURE 43. Low-power microscopic view of recently formed Schmorl's node. There is a defect in the end-plate (above) with extruded nuclear material extending through the defect into the vertebral body (below).

in water content, or degenerative changes; further expansion is also halted by the formation of a cartilaginous or bony shell around the extruded tissue (Figure 44) and the calcification of extruded material (Figure 45).

The cartilaginous "cap" which forms around the extruded tissue is sometimes the result of metaplastic cartilage forming in the marrow at the periphery of the lesion. The extruded material may be surrounded by a zone of increased trabecular bone formation which produces the bony shell limiting further expansion into the vertebral body (Figure 44). The trabeculae forming the walls of these bony shells may exhibit numerous healing trabecular microfractures,[9] indicating that repeated abnormally high stresses are placed on these trabeculae. Frequently there is little or no reactive cartilage or bone formation around the herniation, but the extruded material may be invaded by blood vessels which extend through the gap in the end-plate into the original disc substance. This vascularization of the node and disc may be followed by fibrosis, calcification, or ossification, and will frequently result in radiographically visible changes.

C. Posterior Protrusion: Prolapsed Intervertebral Disc

Much less common than vertical protrusion is posterior protrusion of disc tissue into the spinal canal or posterolateral protrusion into the intervertebral foramina. Posterior protrusion is, however, an important cause of acute and chronic back pain and neurological symptoms. Andrae[25] examined 368 spines at autopsy and found posterior displacements of disc tissue in 56 (15.2%). They were present in 11.5% of male and 18.7% of female spines. About one half of the affected spines showed involvement at several sites, and it was not unusual to find two protrusions affecting a single disc. These observations are in general agreement

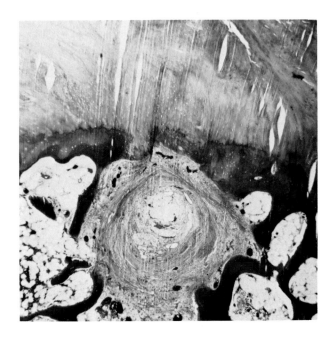

FIGURE 44.   Low-power microscopic view showing bony trabeculae surrounding the extruded nuclear material of a Schmorl's node.

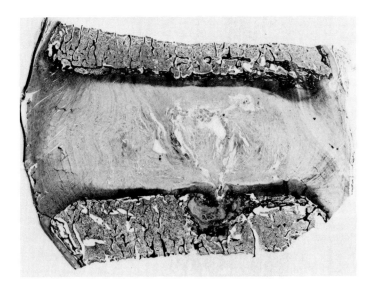

FIGURE 45.   Very low-power microscopic view of section of lumbar disc and
adjacent vertebral bodies in an adolescent. A Schmorl's node has become surrounded by calcification and ossification, which limits its further expansion. Cleft
formation has commenced in the nucleus.

with those of Beadle,[26] who stated that posterior protrusions are present in 15.2% of spines
at autopsy, and Batts,[27] who reported an incidence of 16%. The large majority of posterior
prolapses involve the lumbar and lowest thoracic discs; they less frequently involve the
cervical discs and are rarely present in the thoracic spine. While Andrae[25] did not find any
posterior disc protrusions in any subject less than 30 years old, there have been numerous

observations of posterior protrusions requiring surgical treatment in children, adolescents, and adults below this age.[23,28-30] These findings suggest that disc protrusions in younger persons when the nucleus is still semigelatinous and turgescent are likely to be larger and produce more dramatic symptoms than they would in older persons when the nucleus has become collagenized and has lost its turgescence.

Although a history of preceding trauma may be elicited in many instances, the question remains open as to whether trauma can tear or displace a completely healthy disc, or whether trauma is only the final step in the posterior protrusion of a disc prolapse already in progress. There is no doubt that the discs of the lumbar spine are subjected to severe stresses in everyday life,[24] and it seems likely that fatigue damage, similar to fatigue fractures in bone, could take place in disc tissue when demands surpass functional ability. Schmorl and Junghanns[12] report that early fissure formation and disintegration may be found in discs at an age when the physiology of aging does not explain the disc changes. They are of the opinion that clefts extend in linear fashion posteriorly and posterolaterally to prepare the way for subsequent protrusion. Similar conclusions could be reached from studies of radiation ruptures of the annulus fibrosus.[6,31] These observations are in keeping with the view that most prolapses probably occur before the discs lose their turgescence in middle age, and that discs exhibiting marked degenerative changes in elderly subjects rarely participate in posterior herniations.

Posterior herniations are rarely central in position since the emerging tissue usually tracks around the lateral edge of the posterior longitudinal ligament. Moreover, they are very often situated slightly above or below the central horizontal plane of the affected disc since the emerging tissue also tracks above or below the lateral expansions of the posterior longitudinal ligament, which are firmly attached to the outer layers of the annulus. This explains why sciatic pain and neurological symptoms are commonly unilateral.

During protrusion, either the annulus ruptures completely, or most of the fibers rupture, leaving intact only the outer bands which may bulge markedly into the spinal canal.[23] Thus, fragments of nucleus and annulus may be pushed through the gap. Collins[14] also expressed the opinion that there is seldom a gross breach of the annulus and that the semifluid nuclear material appears to escape by dissecting its way between the fibers. He also stated that some of the inner fibers of the annulus may be fractured, but the outer ones may often be intact and separated rather than ruptured by the herniated nucleus. In contrast, other authors[12,23] state that the prolapsed tissue contains parts of the annulus and cartilage end-plate in addition to nuclear material. However, material removed surgically shortly after a well-documented acute prolapse may show only nuclear material with gelatinous matrix and chordoma-like cells, or mainly fibrocartilage. After a somewhat longer interval, the protrusion shows degenerative changes,[23,32] may become vascularized, organized, chondrified, or even ossi-fied,[14,23,31] and a prominent infiltrate of small lymphocytes may be observed.

Occasionally, large posterior protrusions take the form of small sessile or nipple-shaped swellings covered by the loose extradural areolar tissue of the spinal canal.[8] Ultimately, the shape and size are determined by the bulk and consistency of the extruded material. The presence and severity of pain, and the presence or absence of neurological symptoms depend on the size and direction of the protrusion, but posterolateral prolapses extending into the intervertebral foramina are the type that usually produce the characteristic clinical picture of disc prolapse with sciatica.

Experiments on cadavers and examinations made during surgical exploration of disc prolapses have shown that some protrusions alternately project into the spinal canal and retreat into the disc substance during certain spinal movements, whereas other protrusions are fixed within the canal. Whatever the type of protrusion, its expansion is eventually halted at some stage by a combination of factors which include vascularization and fibrosis, loss of turgescence by the nucleus, and a reduction in physical stresses on the disc by inhibition of movement for reasons of altered mechanics and the presence of pain. These factors produce the circumstances favorable for healing and stabilization of the prolapse to take place. Following vascularization and fibrosis, a reduction in the bulk of the prolapse may follow due to cicatrization. Alternatively, the protrusion may become calcified or ossified and become visible radiographically. However, this healing process is not necessarily accompanied by a relief of symptoms because it is dependent upon the size and location of the prolapse, the degree of spinal rigidity achieved, and other changes in adjacent structures. Moreover, it is not certain whether an arrested prolapse may later enlarge by proliferation of the organizing connective tissues or become the site for repeated episodes of prolapse punctuated by episodes of quiescence.

Probably the most important factor concerned in stabilizing a disc prolapse is the formation of osteophytes encasing the prolapsed tissue as a result of periosteal elevation or some nonspecific irritation.[10] These posterior vertebral body osteophytes occur much less frequently than those commonly seen on the anterolateral margins of the vertebral bodies. When osteophytes form as a result of posterior midline protrusions, they are rarely large enough to significantly narrow the lumbar spinal canal. However, when they form posterolaterally in relation to the intervertebral foramina, they may alone, or together with the prolapsed disc tissue, produce pressure effects on the spinal nerves and give rise to symptoms similar to those caused by disc prolapse alone. Pressure on the nerves may also be aggravated by osteophytes projecting into the intervertebral foramina from the margins of osteoarthritic apophyseal joints (Figure 46). Contributing to the stabilization of the segment at which a posterior protrusion has occurred and to the development of the osteophytes is the thinning of the affected disc (which occurs in many cases[10,23]) or of the discs at adjacent levels.[33]

D. Anterior Protrusions

Anterior and anterolateral protrusions are the rarest of all nuclear protrusions, found in 6% of spines examined by Batts,[34] and probably are the least important from a clinical standpoint. The protruded material shows microscopic features similar to those observed in posterior protrusion (Figure 47)[23] and may become encased by osteophytes at a later stage (Figure 48).[10] Generalized anterior bulging of the whole of the disc substance associated with marginal osteophyte formation is a universal feature of advanced spondylosis of the lumbar spine.

IV. INFECTION, DISCOGRAPHY, AND CHEMONUCLEOLYSIS

A. Clinical

Being largely an avascular structure, the normal disc has been widely considered as being resistant to bacterial invasion or proliferation, but recent studies challenge the validity of that assumption. Infection of the disc can be secondary to involvement of the vertebral bodies by osteomyelitis or result from any procedure contaminating the disc. One cause of disc infection is disc excision; the incidence of this complication is estimated to be 1 to 2.8%.[35,36] While disc infection following radiological discography with contrast material has been considered to be a rare complication and with some investigators attributing it to a chemical or aseptic reaction,[37-41] recent studies have reported an incidence of discitis following this procedure of 1 to 3.4%.[42-44] A recent experimental study has strongly suggested that all cases of discitis following discography with contrast material are due to bacteria introduced at the time of injection.[45] Infective discitis occasionally may ensue after chemonucleolysis with chymopapain.[46] While its rarity has been ascribed to the bactericidal effect of chymopapain, recent experimental studies indicate that chymopapain has little bactericidal effect in vivo.[47]

The hallmark of disc infection usually is severe pain and marked muscle spasm which

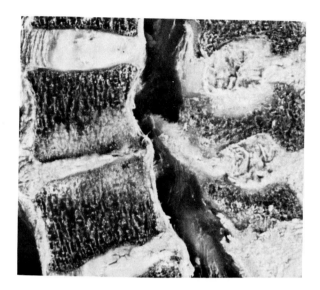

FIGURE 46. Photograph of portion of bisected lumbar spine showing marked thinning of a disc due to a longstanding posterior protrusion. New bone (appearing pale in photograph) has formed in the vertebral bodies above and below, and osteophytes, formed around the protrusion posteriorly, project into the spinal canal. The spinal canal is further narrowed by osteophytes extending from the posterior intervertebral joints which have developed osteoarthritis at the level of the prolapsed disc. (From Vernon-Roberts, B., *The Lumbar Spine and Back Pain*, Jayson, M. I. V., Ed., Churchill Livingston, London, 1987. With permission.)

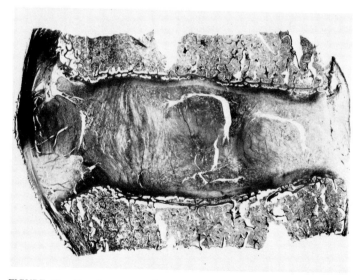

FIGURE 47. Very low-power microscopic view of section of lumbar disc and adjacent vertebral bodies. This shows a rare anterior protrusion of the nucleus with a discrete nodule of protruded nuclear material lying just deep to the anterior longitudinal ligament on the left of the micrograph.

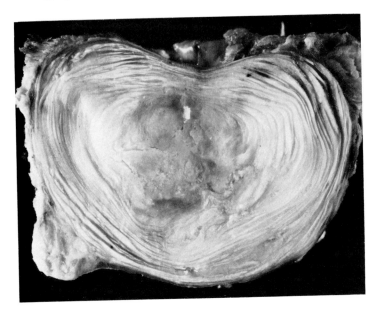

FIGURE 48.   Surface of horizontally divided lumbar disc in a 55-year-old individual. A single large osteophyte is present at the lower left of the photograph at the site of a longstanding anterolateral protrusion.

may have its onset several months postoperatively, or postoperative pain which does not disappear but increases. Radiographic signs include dissolution of the bony end-plate, a progressive loss of disc space height, and a sclerotic bony reaction. Fusion of the vertebral bodies often takes place.

B. Pathology

The histological features following infection of the disc (discitis) show a spectrum of changes similar to those seen in other inflamed tissues of the body. To some extent, depending upon the causative organism and the duration since onset, there is disc vascularization, mature granulation tissue formation in both discs and vertebral bodies, destruction of the cartilage and bony end-plates, vertical disc protrusions in the presence of more marked histological changes, and a constant chronic inflammatory cell infiltrate with the occasional presence of acute inflammatory cells.[44]

Discitis occurring after radiologically normal discography produces large discrete vertical protrusions, while the end-plate lesions following clinical discography tend to be more diffuse.[44] This difference may relate to the high incidence of a prior state of vascularization and the frequent extension of vessels into the cartilage end-plate in radiologically abnormal discs.

Disc space infection following discography with contrast material and after chemonucleolysis with chymopapain has been studied experimentally.[45,47] As in clinical experience,[44] it was found in a sheep model that bacteria are not recoverable from the disc by the time bony end-plate erosions are demonstrable on plain radiographs. The observations on human and experimental material suggest, therefore, that, while bacteria (even in very small numbers) are required to initiate discitis, the destructive inflammatory process still proceeds following the eradication of the causative organisms.

Disc material that infrequently becomes available for histological examination after chemonucleolysis has been attempted by the intradiscal injection of chymopapain, in the absence of infection shows loss of disc space height, cystic cavitation, and cleft formation in the nucleus pulposus. Degenerative changes sometimes are present also affecting the inner annulus. In contrast to the events following disc infection, the end-plates remain intact, and inflammatory cells and granulation tissue are absent from the disc; an occasional finding is the presence of small amounts of granulation tissue and small groups of chronic inflammatory cells in the bone marrow space immediately adjoining the intact end-plates. These latter features, observed in both human and experimental animal spines following the intradiscal injection of chymopapain,[47] are consistent with diffusion taking place across the central region of the end-plate.[11]

It has been reported that, following the intradiscal injection of chymopapain, there may sometimes be radiological evidence of the later restoration of disc space height. In the absence of disc tissue being available for examination in such circumstances, the pathological basis for this phenomenon remains speculative. However, similar to the rare reports of radiological reappearance of the joint space in advanced osteoarthritis, the restoration of disc height following chymopapain injection may result from the formation of fibrous tissue or fibrocartilage.

V. NEOPLASIA — CLINICAL AND PATHOLOGY

With the exception of myelomas, which may sometimes be expected to originate in the vertebral bone marrow (they very frequently involve the spine as part of a generalized malignancy), primary neoplasms of the spine are rare. The very rare tumor, the chordoma, has a peak incidence after the 3rd decade, and has been considered to arise from normal products of the notochord, the nuclei pulposi, or from abnormal nests of primitive notochordal tissue. The tumor is locally invasive and destructive, and rarely metastasizes to distant sites.

In contrast with the rarity of primary neoplasms in the spine, metastatic spread of carcinomas from primary sites elsewhere in the body (particularly lung, breast, prostate, bladder, and thyroid) to the vertebral bodies is exceedingly common. While the destruction and collapse of vertebral bodies frequently ensues, the intervertebral discs are highly resistant to neoplastic invasion; however, disruption of the discs may occur following the collapse of a vertebral body. The resistance of the discs to invasion, even by aggressive, rapidly growing tumors, has been speculatively related to factors normally present in the disc which inhibit the ingrowth of blood vessels upon which the tumor tissue depends for its nutrition. While this may be a contributing factor, other mechanisms may operate in preventing tumor establishment, since the lumbar discs of older individuals frequently show evidence of vascularization in association with the advanced changes of spondylosis.

VI. SPONDYLITIS

A. Clinical
There is a complicated overlapping relationship between spondylitis (inflammation of the spine), inflammation of the sacroiliac joints, peripheral arthritis, chronic inflammatory gastrointestinal diseases, psoriasis, and inflammatory lesions in various organs. There is a hereditary element in most of the clinical features, most marked in patients with obvious spondylitis, who possess the inherited antigenic marker HLA B27 in about 90% of cases, compared with some 10% in healthy white populations. While spondylitis may present at any age, symptoms begin commonly between 17 and 25 years and seldom after 45 years. At the onset of spinal symptoms, a few patients will already have had peripheral arthritis, and some may have had Reiter's disease, psoriasis, or chronic inflammatory bowel disease. In the majority, the first symptoms are spinal or pelvic. Ankylosing spondylitis, the commonest type of spondylitis, typically may result in progressive restriction of spinal movement, spreading from below upward over a period of years. Radiologically, sacroiliitis has been

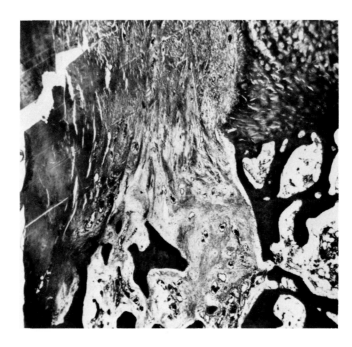

FIGURE 49.   Low-power microscopic view of anterior rim region of a vertebral body in ankylosing spondylitis. The anterior longitudinal ligament is shown on the left of the micrograph. There has been extensive destruction of the end-plate and rim region and their replacement by vascular and granulation tissue.

a cornerstone of early diagnosis. While the detection of the characteristic syndesmophytes *(vide infra)* leading to bony union of adjoining vertebral bodies is pathognomonic of the later phases, destructive lesions of the vertebrae and discs (spondylodiscitis) may be observed as the disease progresses.

B. Pathology

There have been sporadic descriptions[48] of the macroscopic and microscopic changes of the intervertebral discs in ankylosing spondylitis derived from the infrequent cases which come to autopsy during the early or active phases of the disease. Current concepts of the evolution of the disc pathology are derived largely from several studies.[48-50]

It appears that the initial lesion is the site of the anterior and anterolateral attachment of the annulus to the marginal rim of the vertebral body, where there is an infiltrate of chronic inflammatory cells associated with erosive destruction of the adjoining vertebral body bone (Figure 49). Later, the erosive lesions at the attachment of the annulus may heal by the deposition of new bone. This new bone, in continuity with the bone of the marginal rim of the vertebra, extends progressively around the outer fibers of the annulus (Figure 50). These outgrowths of new bone extending vertically are termed syndesmophytes to distinguish them from the vertebral body osteophytes of spondylosis which extend laterally. Moreover, unlike osteophytes, which rarely fuse, the syndesmophytes of adjoining vertebral bodies in ankylosing spondylitis commonly undergo bony union as the syndesmophytes meet to encase the affected discs with bone (Figure 51). The outcome of this process of anterior spondylitis in ankylosing spondylitis is, therefore, the progressive union of vertebral bodies by smooth-surfaced bone (Figures 52 and 53; giving rise to the characteristic bamboo spine in radiology), which contrasts sharply with the outwardly projecting rough and flangelike osteophytes of spondylosis.

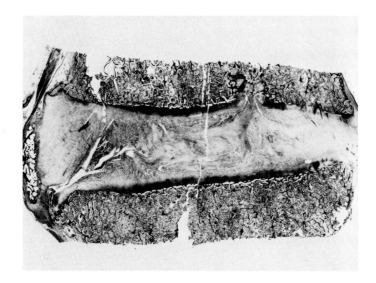

FIGURE 50. Very low-power microscopic view of section of lumbar disc and adjacent vertebral bodies in established ankylosing spondylitis. There is an anterior syndesmophyte underlying the anterior longitudinal ligament (left). The syndesmophyte has almost formed a bridge between the two vertebral bodies. A Schmorl's node also is present.

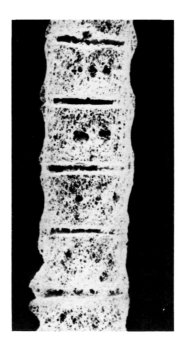

FIGURE 51. Portion of coronally divided macerated lumbar spine in longstanding ankylosing spondylitis. Bony union has taken place between the vertebral bodies at the margins of the discs such that the spine has become rigid.

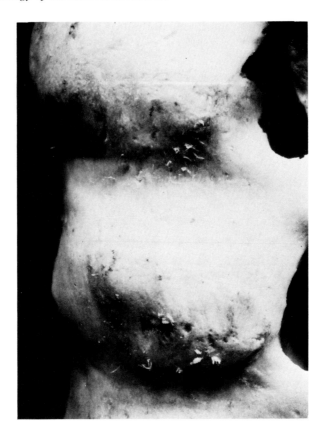

FIGURE 52.   Surface of macerated lumbar spine from patient with longstanding ankylosing spondylitis. There is smooth ossification encasing the discs.

In addition to the changes involving the annulus fibrosus, radiology sometimes reveals evidence of destructive lesions of the end-plates late in the course of ankylosing spondylitis.[50] The basis for these destructive lesions appears to be an inflammatory process causing localized or generalized destruction of the end-plate, accompanied by vertical nuclear protrusions with some localized lesions, and replacement of the disc-bone border rim by granulation tissue and scanty inflammatory cells in extensive lesions. Eventually, the vertebral limits of the destructive process are demarcated by a zone of sclerotic new bone.

Another pathological feature is the presence, late in the course of ankylosing spondylitis, of bridges of bone crossing the central nuclear region of the discs and uniting the adjoining vertebral bodies (Figures 54 and 55), but without narrowing of the disc space height.[51] While in some instances these bridges of bone may represent the end result of the healing of destructive end-plate lesions described above, there appears to have been no destruction of the bony end-plate in some cases. The pathological basis of these transdiscal bone bridges, not previously described, remains speculative.

VII. RHEUMATOID SPONDYLITIS

A. Clinical

Rheumatoid arthritis is a common disease, affecting females more frequently than males, and may begin at any age. In its fully developed form, rheumatoid arthritis is a peripheral, symmetrical, inflammatory disease of synovium which leads to destructive changes in the

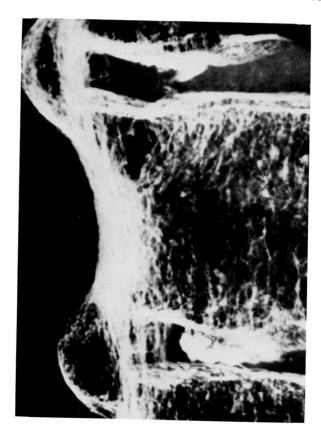

FIGURE 53.   Slab radiograph of portion of lumbar spine from patient with longstanding ankylosing spondylitis. Shows the union of the vertebral bodies by the syndesmophytes encasing the discs.

joints and is associated with the presence of autoantibodies in the blood. Although arthritis is the most prominent manifestation of the disease, it is a generalized disease commonly accompanied by fever, weight loss, anemia, lymph node enlargement, and a wide range of other systemic features. Unlike ankylosing spondylitis and related conditions, rheumatoid arthritis is associated with an increased frequency of the inherited antigenic marker HLA-DRw4, which is present in over 50% of affected individuals.

In addition to disorganization of the atlanto-axial joint by inflammatory erosions, and inflammation and destruction of apophyseal joints, spondylitis in adult rheumatoid arthritis is a common cause of cervical instability and dislocation. Lesions of the thoracic and lumbar spine are relatively uncommon, and sacroiliitis is not a feature of rheumatoid arthritis.

B. Pathology

The destructive lesions of the cervical discs are related to rheumatoid inflammation of the neurocentral joints (uncovertebral joints and joints of Luschka).[49] Neurocentral joints are formed by a cleft in the lateral margin of the disc which lies between the lower lateral border of the vertebral body above and the neurocentral lip of the subjacent vertebra. The cleft is covered laterally by a fibrous membrane lined by synovium. The neurocentral joints are not present at birth, and their appearance depends on the development of the neurocentral lip, which is not completed until about the age of 20 years.[52] When the synovium of the neurocentral joints becomes inflamed, the inflammatory process spreads to erode the adjoining annulus and its attachments, and to some degree the subjacent bone. The eroding granulation tissue spreads around the disc-bone border, usually posteriorly at first.

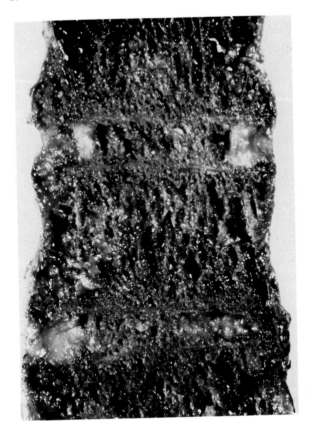

FIGURE 54. Photograph of portion of coronally bisected lumbar spine in ankylosing spondylitis showing numerous bony bridges traversing the discs and uniting the vertebrae above and below.

That rheumatoid cervical disc lesions result from an erosive process arising in the neurocentral joints is consistent with the predominant cervical localization of rheumatoid spondylitis in adults (neurocentral joints) and the rarity of destructive lesions in the cervical discs in the juvenile form of rheumatoid disease.[53]

The involvement of the thoracic or lumbar discs by pathological processes specific to rheumatoid arthritis is rare. A pathological study of the thoracic spine in rheumatoid arthritis[54] has shown that rheumatoid involvement of the costovertebral joints in the thoracic spine may spread to involve the contiguous discs as a destructive inflammatory process with occasional rheumatoid nodule formation. Destructive erosive changes affecting the lumbar discs and adjoining vertebral bodies have been noted radiographically.[55] This author has observed six lumbar spines which showed radiographic evidence of anterior erosions of the vertebral rim subsequently shown pathologically to be due to the presence of rheumatoid nodule-type structures and vascular granulation tissue in the region of the annular attachments (Figure 56).[56] A single patient with similar features has been reported elsewhere.[57] The erosive process appears to affect a larger area of the rim and contiguous lateral border of the affected vertebral body than is the case in ankylosing spondylitis, and may also involve the anterior longitudinal ligament.

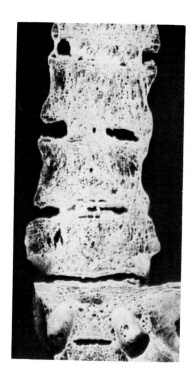

FIGURE 55. Portion of macerated lumbar spine and sacrum in patient with longstanding ankylosing spondylitis. There is union of vertebrae through central bridging and peripheral syndesmophytes.

VIII. DIFFUSE IDIOPATHIC SKELETAL HYPEROSTOSIS (DISH): ANKYLOSING HYPEROSTOSIS AND FORESTIER'S DISEASE

A. Clinical

This condition is present in at least 5% of spines after middle age.[58] It is often asymptomatic, but sometimes is associated with increasing back pain experienced over many years. It is now appreciated that the spinal changes frequently are associated with new bone formation in extraspinal sites, such as the iliac crests, the hip joints, the frontal region of the skull, and elsewhere. It has not been shown to bear a relationship to a specific HLA antigen, and there is conflicting opinion regarding an association with diabetes mellitus. It rarely results in major disability but, particularly in the Japanese, may result in cervical cord compression owing to new bone formation in the posterior longitudinal ligament. Radiologically, the established condition may be readily distinguished from spondylosis and ankylosing spondylitis by its predilection for the cervical and thoracic regions, the sparing of the left side of the spine relative to the right, the preservation of disc-space height, "flowing" or "candle-wax" ossification down the front of the vertebral bodies, and "candle-flame" osteophytes projecting upward from the anterolateral margins of the vertebral rim.

B. Pathology

Macroscopically, there is evidence of new bone formation at the margins and anterior surfaces of the vertebral bodies, particularly on the right side (Figures 57 and 58), which is seen best in macerated specimens.

Histological studies[58] have suggested that the initial event may be a predominantly right-sided anterolateral extension of fibrous tissue in continuity with the annulus fibrosus. This

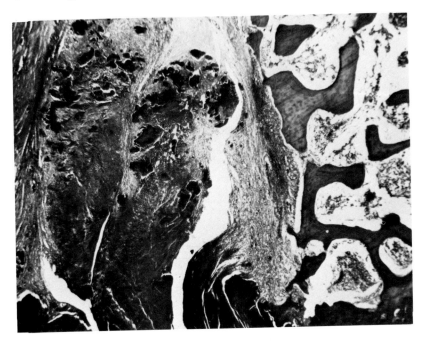

FIGURE 56.   Low-power microscopic view of the anterior region of a lumbar vertebra of a patient with rheumatoid arthritis. The anterior longitudinal ligament is on the left of the field. There is an extensive destructive erosion involving the anterior surface and rim of the vertebral body (right) with the presence of abundant dark-appearing necrotic fibrin-like material (center).

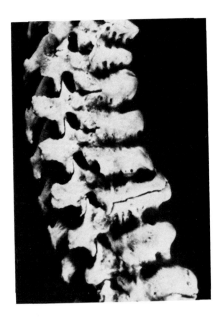

FIGURE 57.   View of portion of right side of macerated thoracic spine in patient with DISH showing the extensive new bone formation which has occurred on the surfaces of the vertebral bodies and around the discs.

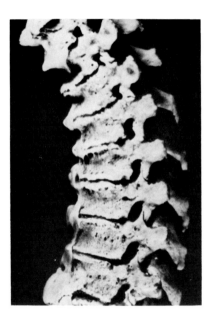

FIGURE 58.   View of left side of spine shown in Figure 57
showing sparing of left side of spine by new bone formation.

process may be inhibited on the left side by the presence of the descending thoracic aorta. The T-shaped or Y-shaped nature of the fibrous tissue extending from the annulus suggests that the tissue extends upward and downward due to the presence of the periosteum covering the surface of each vertebral body. Since elevation of periosteum leads to underlying new bone formation, this could explain the particular flange-shaped (and "candle-flame" radiological appearance) of the marginal osteophytes (Figure 59) and the accretion of new bone on the right anterolateral surface of each vertebral body (Figure 60). While bony ankylosis may result from the fusing of osteophytes, this occurs much less frequently than clinical radiographs suggest. While Schmorl's nodes are present with high frequency,[58] normal disc thickness usually is retained in the advanced condition and may be related to the marked spinal osteoporosis, which is often present.

An increase in the vascularity of the outer annulus has been noted in association with early osteophyte formation in this condition,[58] and it could be speculated that this is compatible with the requirement for the fibrous tissue proliferation and new bone formation.

It is of interest that the spine in DISH has radiological and pathological similarities to the spine in acromegaly. Thus, in acromegaly there is osteophytosis which sometimes extends to bony bridging, accretion of bone which increases the width of the vertebral bodies, and an anterolateral extension of disc tissue with the retention or increase of disc thickness and the absence of disc degeneration.[59,60] There is, however, no other evidence to support an association between acromegaly and DISH.[58,61]

IX. CALCIFICATIONS, DEPOSITIONS, AND PIGMENTATIONS — CLINICAL AND PATHOLOGY

Deposition of calcium salts in the intervertebral discs takes several forms, but is rarely associated with clinical symptoms. The causes of disc calcifications have variously been attributed to degeneration, trauma, hemorrhage, excessive stress, metabolic disturbances, inflammation, or infection.[12] It has been reported that calcification was present in the annulus in 71% and in the nucleus in 6.5% of spines examined pathologically, and that the incidence

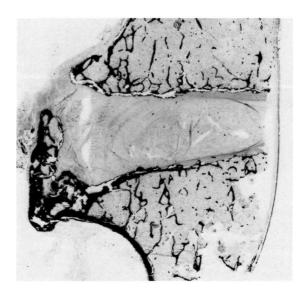

FIGURE 59.   Very low-power microscopic view of section of lumbar disc and adjacent vertebral bodies. Shows a large "candle-flame" osteophyte (left) which has formed on the anterior rim of the lower vertebral body in a patient with DISH.

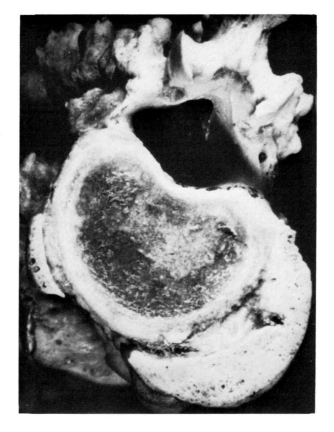

FIGURE 60.   Photograph of horizontal section through macerated thoracic spine in patient with DISH. The manner in which the new bone forms on the outer surface of the vertebral bodies can clearly be seen.

of calcification of the nucleus increases with age.[12] The experience of others, including this author, is that disc calcification is uncommon. In the nucleus, the calcium salt deposition is usually present in cavities in the nucleus, and in small fissures or areas of necrosis of the annulus.[12] However, calcification may sometimes involve the whole of the disc.

Calcium salt deposition may occur in the spine occasionally in the condition of pyrophosphate arthropathy (chondrocalcinosis and pseudogout) in which crystals of calcium pyrophosphate dihydrate (CPPD) are present in articular cartilage, fibrocartilage, synovial tissues, and synovial fluid. While the condition usually is of unknown etiology, it occurs in association with hyperparathyroidism, hemochromatosis, hypophosphatasia, or true gout. The incidence is increased also among patients with acromegaly, Wilson's disease, and diabetes.

When the condition affects the spine, the radiological calcification of the nuclei is due to CPPD cyrstals deposited in the nucleus.

While there have been numerous cases reported of the condition, ochronosis (alkaptonuria) is an extremely rare hereditary metabolic anomaly in which the lack of an enzyme results in the degradation of certain amino acids only to homogentisic acid. The homogentisic acid accumulates in chondroid tissues and ligaments, which are stained brown to black in color. The deposition in the disc is associated with degenerative changes, secondary calcification and ossification of the disc, and the rapid progression of spondylosis-type changes.

Amyloid is the name given to a group of abnormal fibrillar proteins which have a specific affinity for the Congo red stain, after the uptake of which the amyloid material exhibits characteristic green dichroism under polarized light microscopy. (See also Volume I, Chapter 8, Section IV.) It may occur as a primary disease, or may be associated with B cell malignancies, chronic inflammatory disease such as rheumatoid arthritis or tuberculosis, and senescence. It has been reported recently that the deposition of amyloid (not including AA amyloid) occurs in the discs with increasing frequency after the 2nd decade, such that it is present in over 50% of spines during the 4th decade and nearly 90% in the 7th decade.[62] It is of interest to note that the same authors have observed amyloid deposition in the intervertebral discs of a new inbred strain of senescence-accelerated mouse.[63] In a single case of primary amyloidosis, it has been reported that diffuse intervertebral disc calcification occurred.[64]

X. CONCLUSIONS

The intervertebral disc may be primarily or secondarily involved in various pathological processes. It should not be overlooked, however, that, while the disc is a major structural component of the vertebral column, the articulation of the vertebral bodies is accomplished by the three-joint complex comprising the disc and the two apophyseal joints at the same level. Thus, pathological changes in the disc always are accompanied or followed by changes in the apophyseal joints and vice versa. Similarly, disc pathology sometimes may be associated with important changes in the vertebral bodies or ligamentous structures. It has been beyond the scope of this chapter, however, to describe in any detail the important pathology which may be present in structures other than the disc.

REFERENCES

1. **Saunders, J. B. M. and Inman, B. T.,** Pathology of the intervertebral disc, *Arch. Surg. (Chicago),* 40, 389, 1940.
2. **Coventry, M. B., Ghormley, R. K., and Kernohan, J. W.,** The intervertebral disc: its microscopic anatomy and pathology. II. Changes in the intervertebral disc concomitant with age, *J. Bone Jt. Surg.,* 27-A, 233, 19845.

3. **Eckert, C. and Decker, A.,** Pathological studies of intervertebral discs, *J. Bone Jt. Surg.,* 29-A, 447, 1947.

4. **Friberg, S. and Hirsch, C.,** Anatomical and clinical studies on lumbar disc degeneration, *Acta Orthop. Scand.,* 19, 222, 1950.

5. **Harris, R. I. and Macnab, I.,** Structural changes in the lumbar intervertebral discs. Their relationship to low back pain and sciatica, *J. Bone Jt. Surg.,* 36-B, 304, 1954.

6. **Hirsch, C. and Schajowicz, F.,** Studies on structural changes in the lumbar annulus fibrosus, *Acta Orthop. Scand.,* 22, 184, 1953.

7. **Ritchie, J. H. and Fahrni, W. H.,** Age changes in lumbar intervertebral discs, *Can. J. Surg.,* 13, 65, 1970.

8. **Vernon-Roberts, B.,** Pathology of degenerative spondylosis, in *The Lumbar Spine and Back Pain,* Jayson, M. I. V., Ed., Sector, London, 1976, chap. 4.

9. **Vernon-Roberts, B. and Pirie, C. J.,** Degenerative changes in the intervertebral discs of the lumbar spine and their sequelae, *Rheumatol. Rehabil.,* 16, 13, 1977.

10. **Vernon-Roberts, B.,** The pathology and interrelation of intervertebral disc lesions, osteoarthrosis of the apophyseal joints, lumbar spondylosis and low back pain, in *The Lumbar Spine and Back Pain,* 2nd ed., Jayson, M. I. V., Ed., Pitman Medical, Tunbridge Wells, England, 1980, chap. 4.

11. **Urban, J. P. G., Holm, S., Maroudas, A., and Nachemson, A.,** Nutrition of the intervertebral disk. An in vivo study of solute transport, *Clin. Orthop. Relat. Res.,* 129, 101, 1977.

12. **Schmorl, G. and Junghanns, H.,** *The Human Spine in Health and Disease,* Grune & Stratton, New York, 1971.

13. **Hilton, R. C. and Ball, J.,** Vertebral rim lesions in the dorsolumbar spine, *Ann. Rheum. Dis.,* 43, 302, 1984.

14. **Collins, D. H.,** *The Pathology of Articular and Spinal Diseases,* Edward Arnold, London, 1949, chap. 17.

15. **Kirkaldy-Willis, W. H., Wedge, J. H., Yong-Hing, K., and Reilly, J.,** Pathology and pathogenesis of lumbar spondylosis and stenosis, *Spine,* 3, 319, 1978.

16. **Crock, H. V.,** A reappraisal of intervertebral disc lesions, *Med. J. Aust.,* 1, 983, 1970.

17. **Venner, R. M. and Crock, H. V.,** Clinical studies of isolated disc resorption in the lumbar spine, *J. Bone Jt. Surg.,* 63-B, 491, 1981.

18. **Farfan, H. F.,** Effects of torsion on the intervertebral joints, *Can. J. Surg.,* 12, 336, 1969.

19. **Epstein, B. S.,** *The Spine: A Radiological Text and Atlas,* Lea & Febiger, Philadelphia, 1976, 237.

20. **Hilton, R. C., Ball, J., and Benn, R. T.,** Vertebral end-plate lesions (Schmorl's nodes) in the dorsolumbar spine, *Ann. Rheum. Dis.,* 35, 127, 1976.

21. **Schmorl, G.,** Uber die an den Wirbelbandscheiben Vorkommenden Ausdehnungs — und Zerrisungsvorgange und die Dadurch an ihnen und der Wirbelspongiosa Hervorgerufenen Veranderungen, *Verh. Dtsch. Pathol. Ges.,* 22, 250, 1927.

22. **Putschar, W.,** Zur Kenntniss der Knorpelinseln in den Wirbelkorpern, *Beitr. Pathol. Anat.,* 79, 150, 1927.

23. **Coventry, M. B., Ghormley, R. K., and Kernohan, J. W.,** The intervertebral disc: its microscopic anatomy and pathology. III. Pathological changes in the intervertebral disc, *J. Bone Jt. Surg.,* 27-A, 460, 1945.

24. **Nachemson, A.,** Lumbar intradiscal pressure, in *The Lumbar Spine and Back Pain,* 2nd ed., Jayson, M. I. V., Ed., Pitman Medical, Tunbridge Wells, England, 1980, chap. 12.

25. **Andrae, R.,** Uber Knorpelknotchen am hintereb Ende der Wirbelbandscheiben im Bereiche des Spinalkanals, *Beitr. Pathol. Anat.,* 82, 464, 1929.

26. **Beadle, O.,** The intervertebral discs, Medical Research Council, Spec. Rep. Ser. No. 161, Her Majesty's Stationery Office, London, 1931, 161.

27. **Batts, M.,** Etiology of spondylolisthesis, *J. Bone Jt. Surg.,* 21, 879, 1939.

28. **Key, I.,** Intervertebral disc lesions in children and adolescents, *J. Bone Jt. Surg.,* 32-A, 97, 1950.

29. **King, A. B.,** Surgical removal of a ruptured intervertebral disc in early childhood, *J. Pediatr.,* 55, 57, 1959.

30. **Wahren, H.,** Hernie des Nucleus Pulposus bei Einem 12-Jahrigen Kind, *Acta Orthop. Scand.,* 10, 286, 1939.

31. **Lindblom, K. and Hultqvist, G.,** Absorption of protruded disc tissue, *J. Bone Jt. Surg.,* 32-A, 557, 1950.

32. **Deucher, W. G. and Love, J. G.,** Pathologic aspects of posterior protrusions of the intervertebral disks, *Arch. Pathol.,* 27, 201, 1939.

33. **Love, J. G. and Camp, J. D.,** Root pain resulting from intraspinal protrusion of intervertebral discs. Diagnosis and surgical treatment, *J. Bone Jt. Surg.,* 19, 776, 1937.

34. **Batts, M.,** Rupture of the nucleus pulposus. An anatomical study, *J. Bone Jt. Surg.,* 21, 121, 1939.

35. **Ford, L. T. and Key, J. A.,** Postoperative infection of the intervertebral disc space, *South. Med. J.,* 48, 1295, 1955.

36. **Pilgaard, S.,** Discitis (closed space infection) following removal of lumbar intervertebral disc, *J. Bone Jt. Surg.,* 51-A, 713, 1969.

37. **Brodsky, A. E. and Binder, W. F.,** Lumbar discography. Its value in diagnosis and treatment of lumbar disc lesions, *Spine,* 4, 110, 1979.

38. **Collis, J. S. and Gardner, W. J.,** Lumbar discography: an analysis of one thousand cases, *J. Neurosurg.,* 19, 452, 1962.

39. **McCulloch, J. A.,** Chemonucleolysis: experience with 2,000 cases, *Clin. Orthop.,* 146, 128, 1980.

40. **Massie, W. K. and Stevens, D. B.,** A critical evaluation of discography, *J. Bone Jt. Surg.,* 49-A, 1243, 1967.

41. **Wiltse, L. L., Widell, E. H., and Yuan, H. A.,** Chymopapain chemonucleolysis in lumbar disc disease, *J. Am. Med. Assoc.,* 231, 474, 1975.

42. **Fraser, R. D.,** Chymopapain for the treatment of intervertebral disc herniation: the final report of a double-blind study, *Spine,* 9, 815, 1984.

43. **Crock, H. V.,** *Practice of Spinal Surgery,* Springer-Verlag, Vienna, 1983, 52.

44. **Fraser, R. D., Osti, O. L., and Vernon-Roberts, B.,** Discitis after discography. Incidence and pathological findings, *J. Bone Jt. Surg.,* 69-B, 26, 1987.

45. **Fraser, R. D., Osti, O. L., and Vernon-Roberts, B.,** Discitis following discography. An experimental study, *J. Bone Joint Surg.,* 69-B, 31, 1987.

46. **McCulloch, J. A. and MacNab, I.,** *Sciatica and Chymopapain,* Williams & Wilkins, Baltimore, 1983, 203.

47. **Fraser, R. D., Osti, O. L., and Vernon-Roberts, B.,** Discitis following chemonucleolysis. An experimental study, *Spine,* 11, 679, 1986.

48. **Cruickshank, B.,** Lesions of cartilaginous joints in ankylosing spondylitis, *J. Pathol. Bacteriol.,* 71, 73, 1956.

49. **Ball, J.,** Enthesopathy of rheumatoid and ankylosing spondylitis, *Ann. Rheum. Dis.,* 30, 213, 1971.

50. **Cawley, M. I. D., Chalmers, T. M., Kellgren, J. H., and Ball, J.,** Destructive lesions of vertebral bodies in ankylosing spondylitis, *Ann Rheum. Dis.,* 31, 345, 1972.

51. **Vernon-Roberts, B.,** unpublished observations, 1985.

52. **Ecklin, U.,** *Die Altersveranderungen der Halswirbelsaule,* Springer, Berlin, 1960, 17, 28.

53. **Ansel, B. M. and Bywaters, E. G. L.,** Juvenile chronic polyarthritis, in *Copeman's Textbook of the Rheumatic Diseases,* 5th ed., Scott, J. T., Ed., Churchill Livingstone, London, 1978, chap. 14.

54. **Bywaters, E. G. L.,** Thoracic intervertebral discitis in rheumatoid arthritis due to costovertebral joint involvement, *Rheum. Int.,* 1, 83, 1981.

55. **Sims-Williams, H., Jayson, M. I. V., and Baddeley, H.,** Rheumatoid involvement of the lumbar spine, *Ann. Rheum. Dis.,* 36, 524, 1977.

56. **Vernon-Roberts, B.,** unpublished observations, 1976.

57. **Bagenstoss, A. H., Bickel, W. H., and Ward, L. E.,** Rheumatoid granulomatous nodules as destructive lesions, *J. Bone Jt. Surg.,* 34-A, 601, 1952.

58. **Vernon-Roberts, B., Pirie, C. J., and Trenwith, V.,** Pathology of the dorsal spine in ankylosing hyperostosis, *Ann. Rheum. Dis.,* 33, 281, 1974.

59. **Bluestone, R., Bywaters, E. G. L., Hartog, M., Holt, P. J. L., and Hyde, S.,** Acromegalic arthropathy, *Ann. Rheum. Dis.,* 30, 243, 1971.

60. **Jaffe, H. L.,** *Metabolic, Degenerative, and Inflammatory Diseases of Bones and Joints,* Lea & Febiger, Philadelphia, 1972.

61. **Harris, J., Carter, A. R., Glick, E. N., and Storey, G. O.,** Ankylosing hyperostosis. Clinical and radiological features, *Ann. Rheum. Dis.,* 33, 210, 1974.

62. **Takeda, T., Sanada, H., Ishii, M., Matsushita, M., Yamamuro, T., Shimizu, K., and Hosokawa, M.,** Age-associated amyloid deposition in surgically-removed herniated intervertebral discs, *Arth. Rheum.,* 27, 1063, 1984.

63. **Shimizu, K., Ishii, M., Yamamuro, T., Takeshita, S., Hosokawa, M., and Takeda, T.,** Amyloid deposition in intervertebral discs of senescence-accelerated mouse, *Arth. Rheum.,* 25, 710, 1982.

64. **Ballow, S. P., Kahn, M. S., and Kushner, I.,** Diffuse intervertebral disc calcification in primary amyloidosis, *Ann. Intern. Med.,* 85, 616, 1976.

Chapter 12

INFLUENCE OF DRUGS, HORMONES, AND OTHER AGENTS
ON THE METABOLISM OF THE DISC AND THE SEQUELAE
OF ITS DEGENERATION

Peter Ghosh

TABLE OF CONTENTS

I. INTRODUCTION

The growth, maturation, and development of the intervertebral disc, like that of all other connective tissues, are dependent on a variety of extrinsic factors which are known to include nutrients, hormones, and physical stresses. To these ubiquitous determinants can be added other factors such as drugs and biologically active proteins devised by man in an attempt to modify the cellular activity and matrix components of the disc. Although degeneration and structural failure of the disc can be considered to be directly or indirectly responsible for the majority of the clinical problems classified loosely under the heading of back pain, the overall interest in this area has been directed at the development of therapeutic modalities which could be used to suppress the symptoms associated with disc malfunction rather than at the cause. This is particularly evident for the steroidal and nonsteroidal antiinflammatory drugs (AIDs) whose effects on disc cells and the metabolism of matrix components have not been investigated to any significant extent. Since the majority of such agents have been shown in vitro[1-3] and in vivo[4-9] to have suppressive effects on proteoglycan (PG) and collagen synthesis in other connective tissues, it is probable that disc cells would respond similarly. Indeed, the few studies which have been conducted in this area would seem to confirm this view.[10]

In spite of this, clinical trials have been undertaken with such agents, and, while most of the compounds investigated can be said to have questionable therapeutic value, a few would appear to provide some benefit, at least as measured by the relief of patients' symptoms and the support of their return to normal physical activity. In this chapter, an attempt has been made to examine critically this diverse literature and to provide some indications for future developments.

II. NONSTEROIDAL ANTIINFLAMMATORY DRUGS

Nonsteroidal antiinflammatory drugs (NSAIDs) are frequently used in treating the symptoms of back pain. While the origins of this pain may be diverse, as illustrated in Figure 1, common causes are nerve entrapment and inflammation. Inflammation of nerve roots may arise through direct sequestration of disc fragments (which frequently contain fragments of cartilaginous end-plates) into the spinal canal or through irritation of nerve fibers by encroachment of the disc beyond its normal confines.[11] For a detailed discussion of this latter point, the reader is referred to Volume 1, Chapter 5. Under these circumstances there would be every reason to expect that the targeting of NSAIDs to the site of inflammation would be beneficial in suppressing the mediators of pain, in reducing tissue destruction, and in attenuating inflammatory cell recruitment. A prerequisite for such reasoning is that disc tissues, when deposited outside their normal immunologically privileged avascular environment, can engender an antigenic response.

Early experiments to examine this question were undertaken by Bobechko and Hirsch.[12] They used autogenous transplants of nucleus pulposus (NP) placed at vascularized sites of rabbit ears and demonstrated the production of autoantibodies in these animals within 4 days of transplantation. These antibodies were present at the surface of lymphoid cells at primary lymph nodes, where they remained for 3 weeks. Panovich and Korngold[13] employed the mechanical extraction technique of Malawista and Schubert[14] to isolate a PG fraction from the NP of human discs which was then shown to contain at least two antigenic determinants in rabbits. Using the leukocyte migration test, it was subsequently demonstrated[15] that only patients with sequestered disc material could elicit autoantibodies. This finding was confirmed by Gertzbein et al.[16] using 24 patients with well-identified lumbar disc protrusions. A cellular immune response was documented in 72% of these subjects by means of the leukocyte migration inhibition test. At surgery this group showed evidence of sequestered

Pathogenesis of Nerve Root Entrapment Syndromes

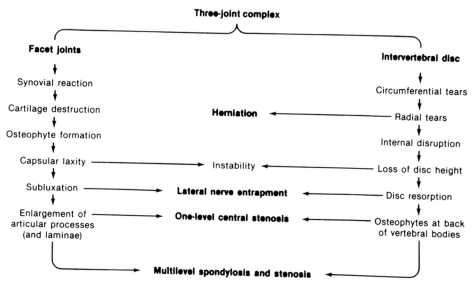

FIGURE 1. The intervertebral disc and the bilateral facet joints constitute a three-joint complex at each spinal level. This figure indicates the spectrum of events that may lead to nerve root entrapment and its sequelae. The progressive changes that occur in the facet joints are listed on the left, those originating from the disc on the right. Together, these may interact, as shown in the center of the figure. In principal, drug intervention could be targeted at any stage of this cascade. In practice, most antiinflammatory agents do not act directly on this process, but suppress the pain and inflammation arising from irritation of nerve roots during disc herniation or sequestration. (From Keim, H. A. and Kirkaldy-Willis, W. H., *Clin. Symp.*, 32(6), 19, 1980. Reproduced by courtesy of CIBA-GEIGY Ltd., Basel, Switzerland. All rights reserved.)

disc material in the spinal canal. However, none of the patients studied showed a positive result in the Ochterlony gel diffusion test confirming the absence of circulating antibodies. In later publications from this group[17,18] the lymphocyte transformation test was added as a means of assessing cellular immunity, and again positive results were obtained only in those individuals in which disc material had escaped from its normal domain.

There is thus good evidence that both degraded and undegraded components of the extracellular matrix of the disc can provoke an inflammatory response when they become exposed to immune-competent cells of the circulation. While extrusion of disc fragments into the spinal canal can clearly be identified as an initiator of an inflammatory reaction, it is also possible that leakage of disc components through a damaged, but intact annulus may be sufficient to promote a response, although the evidence for such a process is presently inadequate.[19] However, it is important to note that not all such events are troublesome, as is demonstrated by the not uncommon clinical experience of positive myelograms in patients who are asymptomatic and the high incidence of protrusions found in cadaveric discs of individuals with no previous history of back pain (see Chapter 11 for a discussion of this point).

Antiinflammatory drug therapy, particularly the local administration of corticosteroids, could, on the immunological grounds described above, be useful in the treatment of the early phase of nerve root inflammation. However, there would be little point in administering such agents for chronic root pain which arises from different causes. Here, intraneural fibrosis may exist as a consequence of chronic inflammation. It has been postulated that this can cause stenosis of nerve roots as well as ischemia.[20] Once the chronic stages of inflammation have been established the process is probably irreversible.

A. Clinical Studies

The number of clinical trials designed specifically to examine the effectiveness of antiinflammatory drugs in suppressing the pain and inflammation associated with disc herniation are few and far between. This is most noticeable for double-blind trials designed to eliminate the possible placebo response which appears to be particularly high for back pain sufferers. In a small double-blind trial consisting of 23 patients diagnosed as having prolapse lumbar discs, Radin and Bryan[21] found that phenylbutazone produced a statistically significant improvement in motor weakness ($p < 0.05$) but had less effect ($p < 0.1$) on straight-leg raising than in the placebo-treated group. The protocol required administering placebo or 600 mg phenylbutazone orally for 2 days and the 300 mg for 8 days. Patients were assessed on a 0 to 3 scale by subjective (sciatica at rest and overall discomfort) and four objective criteria (straight-leg raising, popliteal compression, contralateral pain on straight-leg raising, and motor weakness). From this study, it was concluded that while phenylbutazone provided some improvement in physical signs, it did not decrease the number of patients requiring surgical intervention for disc prolapse. From these data, these authors concluded that administration of phenylbutazone did not modify the course of the disease.

A double-blind comparison of difunisal against paracetamol in the management of chronic back pain has been described.[22] A randomly selected group of 16 patients received diflunisal, and 14 paracetamol. All had displayed symptoms of back pain for many months and, in some cases, years prior to entry into the study. The trial was conducted over 4 weeks using 1000 mg daily of diflunisal and 4000 mg of paracetamol. The response to drug was monitored by both subjective and objective parameters such as pain relief, functional disability, pain on spinal extension, forward bending, and patient self-assessment using an analogue scoring system. After completing the trial period it was found that none of the paracetamol group was free of symptoms, but a proportion of the patients experienced some relief to a varying degree. In contrast the diflunisal-treated group was reported to show improvement, and four of the group continued to use this drug as their sole means of symptomatic relief for 24 to 40 months after completing the trial. As the drug was well tolerated and showed little evidence of adverse side effects, the investigator considered diflunisal to be a safe and effective means of treating low back pain. In the absence of evidence to the contrary, it is likely that the mode of action of diflunisal was primarily due to its strong analgesic properties.

Diflunisal has also been evaluated against naproxen-sodium and placebo in a threeway double-blind crossover trial using 37 patients with chronic back pain.[23] Naproxen-sodium (550 mg) was given twice daily, and diflunisal (500 mg) given at the same frequency for 14 days after admission to the trial with appropriate drug washout periods. Pain was assessed using both visual analogue scales as well as descriptive criteria. Side effects and patient's drug preferences were also monitored. Naproxen-sodium was reported to be superior to placebo in relieving global pain and, depending on the assessment method, was considered beneficial in relieving night pain and pain produced by movement. In contrast to the report of Hickey,[22] this study was not able to demonstrate a statistically significant difference between the diflunisal and placebo groups. Whether this difference in findings was due to the shorter trial period used by Berry et al.[23] or represents a consequence of the different method of patient selection and assessment cannot be readily determined. However, such descrepancies are not uncommon and serve to illustrate the inherent problems of interpreting the outcome of drug trials where the method of patient selection, trial period, and means of determining drug response varies from one investigator to another.

In an attempt to reduce the interpatient variation in a double-blind crossover trial of indomethacin, flurbiprofen, and placebo, patient groups were matched on the basis of their radiologically determined grade of lumbar spondylopathy.[24,25] Twenty-four patients completed the trial, each being allocated to a group of four receiving 300 mg flurbiprofen, 150 mg indomethacin, or placebo daily for 2 weeks followed by crossover using a Latin square sequence to minimize carryover effects. Drug response was assessed by objective measurements which included spinal flexion, a femoral nerve stretch test, and straight-leg raising. Pain, general condition, and side effects were assessed using an analogue scale. Apart from the standard hematological and biochemical blood assessments, patient sera were also monitored during the trial for the levels of total glycosaminoglycan. Statistical analysis of the results showed that flurbiprofen and indomethacin were comparable in their ability to improve patient mobility, but indomethacin was more effective than flurbiprofen in producing pain relief. However, the intensity and frequency of side effects was higher when indomethacin was taken. In general, both drugs produced a better response than the placebo group, but no correlation could be found between the drug regime used and level of serum glycosaminoglycans. This latter finding would suggest that the turnover of disc PGs was not influenced by either of the drugs, although there is some evidence that the measurement of serum glycosaminoglycans does not truly reflect the metabolic status of the disc, for example, during remodeling in scoliosis[26] or chymopapain-produced chemonucleolysis.[27]

Recent studies using monoclonal and polyclonal antibodies to specific regions of the PG molecules have been used with some success to monitor cartilage breakdown in joint diseases such as osteoarthritis[28,29] and rheumatoid arthritis.[30,31] It is possible that such techniques can provide more selective serum markers to follow disc turnover in drug trials of the type described. However, laboratory evidence that any of the currently used drugs can influence disc PG metabolism is still lacking.

A variety of open clinical trials using AID preparations for the management of back pain of diverse etiologies have been described. Since the majority of the these drugs also possess powerful analgesic properties, any useful effects reported from such investigations cannot be exclusively attributed to the suppression of inflammation. Of the NSAIDs examined, including indomethacin,[32-36] oxyphenbutazone,[37] naproxen,[38] flufenamic acid, mefenamic acid,[39] and diclofenac,[40] none can be said to be adequate in relieving all symptoms. This suggests that the present strategies are naive and are in desperate need of revision. Such a situation is open for exploitation, and a miscellaneous collection of preparations have been forwarded as alternatives to the traditional AID described above. While the rationales proposed for such applications are occasionally soundly based, in general, the explanations offered are highly questionable. A summary of the published literature on some of these studies is shown in Table 1, from which it can be seen that colchicine and the free radical scavengers catalase and superoxide desmutase (organotein) emerge as agents of some interest.

B. Colchicine

Rask was the first to report useful effects of colchicine for the management of patients with lower back problems, although the reasons for its selection were not stated.[41] Several papers subsequently appeared using open trial methods;[42,43] the largest describes the results from 500 patients. A rapid and highly positive response ($\geq 70\%$) was reported with complete remission of symptoms in some cases. Others[45] have also reported beneficial results with colchicine using open trial methods. A double-blind clinical trial[45,46] using 60 patients (which 38 completed) reported a positive effect of colchicine, against placebo, for improving muscle spasm, muscle weakness, straight-leg raising, and pain relief at the 99.9% confidence level. The criteria for selecting patients was low back pain with or without leg pain of at least 2 months duration. The authors did not indicate whether all participants in the trial had myelographic evidence of disc prolapse, although the protocol published indicates that these were routinely undertaken. A summary of some of the results obtained in this latest trial[46] are shown in Figure 2. The beneficial effects of colchicine appear exceptionally high and could not be attributed to a placebo response. Nevertheless, the application of this drug has been confined to a limited number of investigators in the U.S., and more extensive independent investigations should be undertaken before its therapeutic worth can be accepted

Table 1
MISCELLANEOUS PREPARATIONS USED IN THE TREATMENT OF DISC DISORDERS

Substance	Diagnosis	No. of patients	Dosage	Trail type	Method of assessment	Response	Rationale	Ref.
Colchicine	Herniated disc disease, damaged disc syndrome	500	0.6—1.2 mg i.v. initially, then 1.2 mg orally daily	Open	Pain, SLR, radiographically, thermography	68% good to excellent	See text	41, 42, 43
Colchicine	Lower back pain	60	1.0 mg i.v. initially, then 0.6 mg orally for 14 days	Double-blind	Pain, SLR, muscle spasm, weakness	Marked and immediate improvement	See text	44, 45, 46
Baclofen	Acute lower back pain	200	30—80 mg orally	Double-blind	Pain, SLR, spinal flexion, muscle spasm	Severe symptoms most relieved (7/9 parameters)	Not discussed	238
Diazepam	Cervical spondylosis, cervical and lumbar disc protrusion	62	6—8 mg orally daily	Open	Improvement scales	66% significant improvement	Muscle relaxant	239
Diazepam	Lumbar spondylosis, disc prolapse	50	40 mg i.m. followed by 8 mg orally	Double-blind	Pain, SLR, spasm, hyperextension	Indistinguishable from placebo	Muscle relaxant	240
Diazepam/ pentabarbital	Disc degeneration	62	6.25—20.0 mg diazepam i.v., 100—200 mg pentabarbital i.v.	Double-blind	As discography premedicant, pain response, vital signs, etc.	Diazepam superior to pentabarbital	Muscle relaxant	241
Chymoral (trypsin/ chymotrypsin)	Sciatica	30	50,000 units orally	Double-blind crossover	Pain, SLR	Significant benefit	Reduction in inflammatory edema of nerve root	242
Chymoral	Lumbar disc prolapse	93	2 tablets 4 × daily, orally (as above)	Double-blind	Pain, SLR, spinal flexion, muscle weakness	Significant reduction and SLR important, but other parameters same as placebo	Reduction in inflammatory edema	243

Urea	Disc herniation, nerve root compression	25	40 g i.v. 1—4 × per day maximum	Open	Pain, SLR symptomatic relief	56—76% reduction in symptoms, 20% complete relief	Reduction in nerve root pressure	244
Dimethyl sulfoxide	Discogenic disease	18	90% aqueous solution applied topically	Open	Subjective and objective responses	50% beneficial response	Irritant effects, hygroscopicity, effects on proteins?	245
Vitamin B_{12}/gangliosides	Postoperative radiculopathy	30	B_{12}, 5000 units i.m.; ganglioside, 40 mg i.m.	Open	Subjective criteria, electromyography, electroneuronography	Improvement in treated group	Neurotropism	246
Catalase	Cervical and lumbar disc degeneration	648	25,000 units i.m. for 10 days, then 3 × weekly	Open	Rate of recovery, ischial syndromes	Accelerated recovery in treated group	Enzymatic decomposition of H_2O_2 to O_2	57
Organotein (superoxide dismutase)	Disc syndromes, spondylosis	154 dogs	2.5 mg subcutaneous for 6 days, then alternate days	Double-blind	Gait impairment, incontinence	72% effective	Removal of superoxide free radicals	

Note: i.v., intravenous; i.m., intramuscular; SLR, straight-leg raising test.

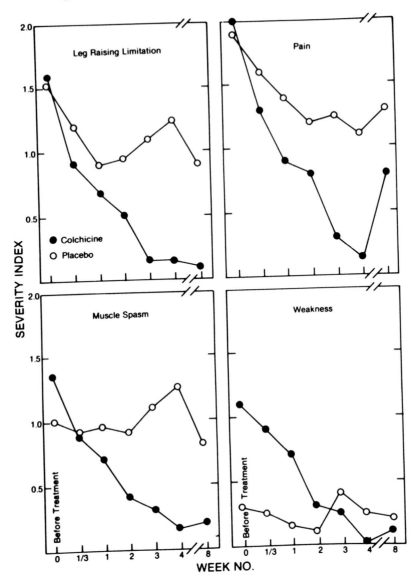

FIGURE 2.   Summary of results reported for a double-blind study of colchicine (-●-●-) against placebo (-○-○-). Thirty-eight patients with resistant disc disorders of at least 2 months' duration participated in this trial, and the results shown were statistically significant at the 99.0% confidence level. Of the 17 in the colchicine-treated group, 3 did not respond, while 14 out of the 21 in the placebo-treated group showed no clinical improvement. (From Meek, J. B. et al., *J. Neurol. Orthop. Med. Surg.*, 6, 211, 1985. With permission.)

unequivocally. Futhermore, colchicine is a highly toxic compound, its LD_{50} in the mouse being about one sixth that of strychnine. Apart from its ability at high dose to induce leukopenia, hyperperistalsis, diarrhea, vomiting, and dehydration, some individuals are highly sensitive to the drug, particularly those with impaired liver and kidney function.[47]

The mechanism of action of colchicine in relieving the symptom of disc disease is presently unknown. However, considerable data have accumulated about this drug due to its use in the treatment of acute gouty arthritis.[47] In this regard, colchicine's action appears to be mediated via its effects on microtubules of cell membranes which are involved in cell motility and in biosynthetic and secretory processes. These and other pathways in which colchicine could influence the symptoms associated with disc protrusion have recently been reviewed by Francis.[48] The target cells in acute gout would appear to be polymorphonuclear leukocytes and phagocytic synoviocytes, both of which participate in the urate crystal-induced inflammation. Polymorphonuclear leukocyte chemotaxis is suppressed by colchicine, and the release of collagenase by stimulated synoviocytes is also modulated. In addition, colchicine also has a multitude of effects on other cellular processes which, without doubt, contribute to its effectiveness in controlling acute gouty arthritis. However, the demonstrated ability of this drug to suppress neutrophile recruitment to the inflammatory site and block intracellular communications following phagocytosis would be expected to be of some benefit in attentuating the inflammation associated with nerve root irritation.[48]

C. Free Radical Scavengers

Polymorphonuclear leukocytes and cells of the monocyte-macrophage lineage are also significant sources of high-energy oxygen-derived free radicals. These inflamogens oxidize polyunsaturated lipids, disrupt liposomal and cellular membranes, and degrade biopolymers such as hyaluronic acid, collagen, and DNA, thereby incurring extensive tissue damage.[49-54] Using animal models of inflammation, McCord and co-workers[55] demonstrated that superoxide desmutase (SOD; in a slow-acting form) provided a useful antiinflammatory effect by catalyzing the conversion of the superoxide free radical (O_2^-) to molecular oxygen and hydrogen peroxide. Catalase, together with the peroxidases, provides a means of removal of hydrogen peroxide within cells by conversion to water and molecular oxygen.[54]

In principle, therefore, scavengers of oxygen-derived free radicals, such as SOD, catalase, glutathione peroxidase, vitamin E, and the iron chelator desferrioxamine, could provide protection to both cells and tissue during inflammatory cell invasion. Whether the reported[56,57] beneficial effect of SOD and catalase in the management of disc degeneration proceeds via the mechanism proposed has yet to be established, but clearly such a rationale is worthy of further investigation.

III. CORTICOSTEROIDS AND HORMONES

Glucocorticosteroids have been employed in the management of inflammatory conditions, including rheumatoid arthritis, for well over 30 years. The success of these agents led to their widespread, and sometimes indiscriminate, use, frequently leading to manifestations of Cushing's syndrome.[58] The pharmaceutical industry, in response to the shortcomings of hydrocortisone, examined many thousands of structural analogues. From these investigations new molecules emerged which reduced mineralocorticoid activity and increased antiinflammatory potency relative to hydrocortisone.[59] Table 2, which compares the properties of some of the more commonly used corticosteroid preparations, illustrates this point.

The manner by which the glucocorticoids may influence the inflammatory processes is wide ranging and extremely complex, and because of the limitation of space can only be briefly reviewed here. However, their profound effects on leukocyte trafficking and function must be considered to be of paramount importance. Corticosteroids induce lymphocytopenia in both experimental animals and man.[60,61] In humans, this is due to the redistribution of lymphocytes (primarily as T cells) from the intravascular compartments to lymphoid tissues and bone marrow[61] (see Figure 3), probably due to cell surface modification.[61,62] Glucocorticosteroids also have profound effects on cells of the monocyte lineage where depletion from blood by a process similar to that for lymphocytes occurs.[61,63] In addition, these agents modify monocyte and macrophage response to chemotactic factors, lymphokine migration inhibition factor (MIF), and macrophage activation factor (MAF;[61-63] Figure 4). An example of how macrophage may respond to a foreign protein and the sites at which glucocorticoids may act is shown in Figure 5. Once activated by T-cell lymphokines, the macrophage can

Table 2
PROPERTIES OF SOME OF THE COMMONLY USED
GLUCOCORTICOIDS

Duration of action of preparation	Antiinflammatory potency	Equivalent dose (mg)	Sodium-retaining potency	Approximate plasma half-life (min)
Short-acting				
Hydrocortisone (cortisol)	1.0	20.00	2+	90
Cortisone	0.8	25.00	2+	30
Prednisone	4.0	5.00	1+	60
Prednisolone	4.0	5.00	1+	200
Methylprednisolone	5.0	4.00	0	180
Intermediate-acting				
Triamcinolone	5.0	4.00	0	300
Long-acting				
Betamethasone	20—30	0.60	0	100—300
Dexamethasone	20—30	0.75	0	100—300

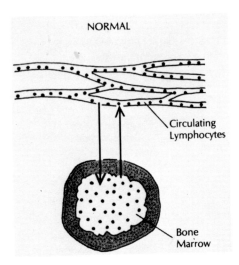 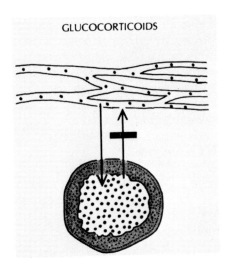

FIGURE 3.   Glucocorticoid-induced lymphocytopenia is due to a temporary redistribution of lymphocytes between vascular and lymphoid tissues and bone marrow. Normally recirculating cells move freely between the blood, lymphatic tissues, and bone marrow. Glucocorticoids enhance the egress of cells from blood vessels to extravascular tissues, particularly bone marrow, and also block their return. Monocytes and eosinophils are similarly affected. (From Claman, N. N., *Hosp. Pract.*, July, 126, 1983. With permission.)

release a variety of metallo and serine proteinases which can influence fibrinolysis and degrade collagen, elastin, and proteoglycans. The glucocorticosteroids can prevent tissue destruction by these processes by blocking the release of macrophage proteinases as shown diagramatically in Figure 5. Finally, glucocorticosteroids are known to prevent adherence of neutrophils to blood vessel walls, thereby reducing their immigration, in response to chemotactic factors, into tissues. One positive effect of margination of these phagocytic cells is a reduction in the number of leukocytes which accumulate at the inflammatory locus. The control of cell trafficking, inhibition of the release of soluble proteins and enzymes implicated in cell activation, and tissue destruction must all be considered as potential pathways on which the glucocorticosteroids could act. While there is no direct evidence that glucocorticosteroids act at inflamed nerve roots in the manner described above, the clinical findings of relief of symptoms would support such a deduction.

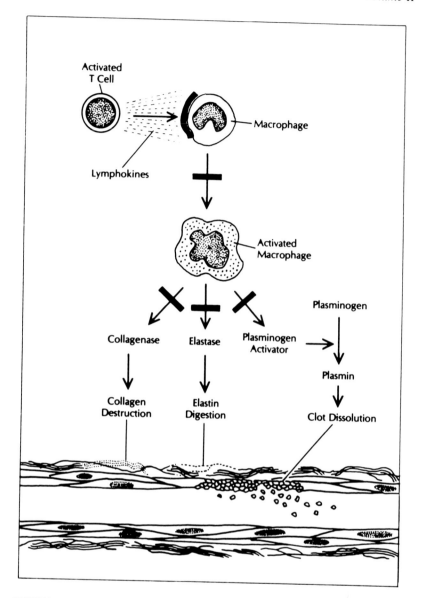

FIGURE 4. Glucocorticoids can prevent tissue destruction associated with inflammation by inhibiting macrophage activation by T lymphocytes and other cells. The secretion of tissue-degrading enzymes, such as collagenases and elastase, as well as plasminogen activator by stimulated macrophages can also be modulated by glucocorticoids. (From Claman, N. N., *Hosp. Pract.*, July, 131, 1983. With permission.)

A. Clinical Studies

In their clinical applications corticosteroids have been used systemically[64-68] and locally[69-77] to suppress the inflammation and pain associated with nerve root irritation or compression arising from disc herniations. Several review articles have appeared on this subject.[78-80] Although Green[66] reported rapid relief of radicular pain due to myelographically proven lumbar disc herniation in 100 patients by intramuscular dexamethasone treatment for 7 days, the general concensus is that local administration of these drugs is preferable to the systemic route. Corticosteroids were used extradurally in the 1960s by Harley[77] and by Gardner and co-workers[69,71,81] in an attempt to reduce adhesions and limit fibrotic tissue

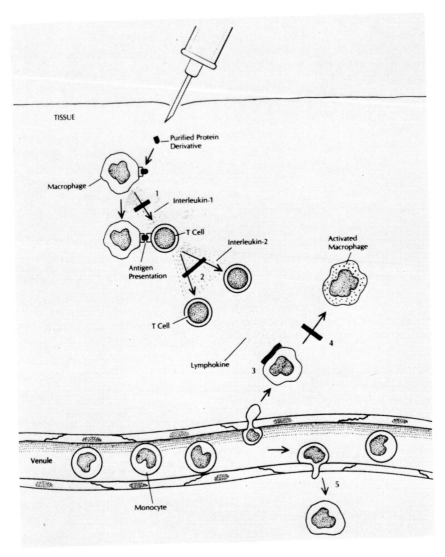

FIGURE 5.   The role of glucocorticoids in the modulation of antigen-induced monocyte recruitment and lymphocyte activation is exemplified using tuberculin as a purified protein derivative (PPD). After the antigen-presenting macrophage picks up PPD, the response is modified by glucocorticoids by (1) blockade of interleukin-1 production by macrophage, (2) blockade of T cell production of interleukin-2, (3) diminished macrophage response to lymphokines, (4) inhibition of macrophage activation, and (5) increased migration of monocytes from blood to tissue distant from the PPD injectionsite. (From Claman, N. N., *Hosp. Pract.*, July, 125, 1983. With permission.)

proliferation at the inflammatory nidus of irritated spinal nerve roots. Good results ($\geq 60\%$) were reported, and several double-blind clinical trials were subsequently undertaken.[82,83] Dilke and co-workers[83] used methylprednisolone extradurally in 100 consecutive patients identified as having nerve root compression. A significant improvement, attributed to the antiinflammatory effect of the drug, was reported. Others using dexamethasone[64] or methylprednisolone[74,75] have obtained less encouraging results, although the latter study[75] was conducted using young adult athletes.

Intraspinal routes of administration of corticosteroids are considered to have the advantages of maintaining a high local concentration of the drug at the inflammatory nidus while minimizing the potential side effects frequently encountered when these agents are used systemically. This rationale may not be entirely valid as, after intrathecal injection of adrenal cortical steroids into dogs, the cerebrospinal fluid levels were found to be no greater than when the same dosage of drug was administered by slow intravenous infusion.[84] Opinion augurs against intrathecal administration, epidural application being considered safer and just as efficacious.[71,73,75,78,79] Insoluble formulations of the corticosteroids are generally administered via this route, thereby achieving a high drug concentration in combination with a long drug half-life. Low aqueous solubility has been achieved not only by structural modification of the steroid to include hydrophobic substituents, but also by utilizing detergents and surfactants to modify the binding and absorption properties of the drug. Depomedrol®, which consists of methyl prednisolone acetate compounded with polyethylene glycol and myristryl-γ-picolinium chloride, is an example of such a preparation. The latter can form micelles in aqueous solution, thus providing a hydrophobic interface for the methyl prednisolone. Because of the irritant effect of the drug vehicle used in Depo-medrol® and several reports of meningitis after its application,[85] its use intrathecally or epidurally is no longer approved by the manufacturer.

Intradiscal administration of hydrocortisone was first reported in 1956 by Feffer.[86] Although the basis for selecting this route was not postulated, a possible pathway for consideration might have been suppression by the steroid of enzyme release by disc cells. Nevertheless, by 1969, 244 patients with severe lumbar disc disease, with and without myelographic defects, had been treated by this route and evaluated after a 4- to 10-year follow-up period.[87] Of these, 46.7% showed a good response with complete or nearly complete remission, whereas 53.3% did not respond. A more detailed analysis of the data indicated that patients in the older age group and those with back pain rather than radicular pain responded more favorably to this mode of treatment.[88]

Graham[89] undertook a double-blind trial comparing chymopapain with intradiscal hydrocortisone using two groups of 20 patients with sciatic pain, some of whom included workers' compensation cases. Not only were the male-female distribution or mean ages of the two groups not matched, but also in some instances two-level (chymopapain or hydrocortisone) injections were used while in others, only one level was treated. The results of this uncontrolled study showed little distinction between the two methods of treatment. Approximately half the groups presented a fair to good response.

Wilkinson and Schuman[90] used multiple intradiscal injections of methylprednisolone acetate suspension (as Depo-medrol®) to treat lumbar and cervical disc disease. A success rate of 52% was reported for 29 patients with lumbar disc disease 1 month after injection. However, this had decreased to 33% after 3 months and 21% after 6 months. A similar result was obtained for 14 patients with cervical disc problems.

From these studies, it is clear that intradiscal corticosteroid treatment produces very little long-term benefit. Since it has been demonstrated that blood vessels enter only the periphery of the normal disc (see Chapter 4), there is no reason to expect inflammatory cells to be present at the sites where the steroid is delivered. However, prolapsed discs may well be invaded by capillaries along annulus clefts caused by herniation and could provide a route of entry of plasma cells to the central regions of the disc (see Chapters 10 and 11 for a detailed discussion of this point). Under such circumstances, intradiscal administration of corticosteroids could be useful in suppressing neutrophil migration and might explain the short-term good response observed in some patients so treated.

B. Experimental Studies

Although the clinical studies described above suggest some useful therapeutic effects for corticosteroids, experimental evidence indicates that this is probably not due to a direct effect on the components of the intervertebral disc. In fact, hydrocortisone would be contraindicated for such a purpose on the basis of the few animal experiments described.

Davidson and Small[91] were the first to undertake experiments to evaluate the effects of hormones on the metabolism of disc components. The in vivo metabolism of the chondroitin sulfate and keratan sulfate of proteoglycans extracted from the NP of mature and immature rabbits was determined by the incorporation into these moeties of radioactivity-labeled glucose. The disc glycosaminoglycans were assessed after acid hydrolysis to release galactosamine and glucosamine, which were then separated on a Dowex®-50 ion exchange column.

Apart from the expected pattern of increased keratan sulfate in the NP with aging (see Volume I, Chapter 6), the half-life of this glycosaminoglycan in the NP of mature animals was found to be considerably longer ($t_{1/2} \sim 120$ days) than the corresponding chondroitin sulfate ($t_{1/2} \sim 3$ to 5 days). While administration to mature animals of growth hormone (0.5 mg/kg, 1.53 units/mg) 7 to 10 days prior to injection of the radioisotope increased the turnover of both chondroitin sulfate and keratan sulfate to levels comparable to the immature group, estrogen-treated female rabbits showed a different response. Estrogen produced little effect on the keratan sulfate pool, but increased the half-life for chondroitin sulfate from 5 to 25 days. Cortisone, at a dosage of 5.0 mg/kg/day, induced only marginal effects on the metabolic half-life of the chondroitin sulfate, but decreased the keratan sulfate turnover from more than 60 days in control animals to about 5 days in the treated group. From these results, it was suggested that cortisone inhibited incorporation of sulfate into newly synthesized glycosaminoglycans. This interpretation was consistant with studies using hyaline cartilage[92-94] and skin.[94,95]

A short histological-histochemical report of the effects of estradiol, testosterone, cortisone acetate, somatotropin, thyrotropin, and parathyroid hormone on the lumbar disc of growing nonchondrodystrophoid dogs has been described.[96] In the low-dose estradiol- or testerone-treated groups, metachromasia of the annulus fibrosus (AF) was observed which progressed to fragmentation at higher doses. A similar but less marked effect was noted for the animals treated with cortisone acetate and somatotropin, while thyrotropin produced annular changes comparable to that seen with the sex hormones. The limited amount of data presented in this study reduces its value, but it does serve to illustrate the profound effect that hormones and steroids may have on the discs of growing animals, particularly with respect to the biosynthesis of matrix components.

Haimovici[97] investigated the effects of repeated administration of adrenocorticotropic hormone (ACTH) on artificially created defects in mature rabbit discs. The defects were produced by transverse incisions (1.5 to 2.0 cm) made into the anterior aspect of lumbar discs so that the NP protruded beyond the AF outer surface. Ten units of ACTH (as ACTH Prolongal, Cortrofina-Z-Organon) were given intramuscularly 3 days after surgery and continued on alternate days thereafter for 4 weeks and then every 3rd day for a 2nd month. Animals were sacrificed and disc tissues examined 13, 26, 39, and 55 days after the initial disc injury. At the dosage level used, ACTH was observed not to influence the cellular activity or repair processes stimulated in the discs by surgical evolution of the NP.

More recently, Higuchi and Abe[10] described a light and electron microscopic study of the NP of mice treated with various doses of hydrocortisone. Animals were treated with 1.0, 5.0, or 10.0 mg/kg of hydrocortisone for 1, 2, or 4 weeks and notochordal cells examined at the center and periphery (the most metabolically active region)[8] of the NP. With low-dose hydrocortisone administration, the cells at the periphery of the NP showed, within 1 week, development of large vacuoles and diminution of the perinuclear matrix. By 2 weeks, the intercellular space had widened, and the cells became clustered. Cell necrosis and degeneration was apparent by 4 weeks. The central region of the NP showed less marked changes than the periphery, but by 4 weeks notochordal cells were clustered and surrounded by a metachromatically stainable matrix. The results obtained at the higher dose of hydrocortisone corresponded to an acceleration of the degenerative processes observed at the lower dose, and again abberations in cells at the periphery of the NP preceded those in the center. From this study it was concluded that notochordal cells responded to corticosteroids by a reduction in metabolic activity leading eventually to cell degeneration.

On the basis of the above studies, as well as the known suppressant effects of corticosteroids on the biosynthesis of PGs and collagen in other connective tissues,[2,4,8,92-95,98,99] it would be reasonable to conclude that chronic administration of corticosteroids has a deleterious effect on the metabolism of disc cells.

C. Diabetic Spondylopathy

The strong association between hyperstotic spondylosis and diabetes mellitis is well known.[100-103] While raised levels of somatotropin in diabetics have been suggested to be implicated, the specific humoral factors responsible for the degenerative changes which take place in the intervertebral disc have not been identified. A histochemical study of inter- vertebral discs of immature Chinese hamsters that spontaneously developed diabetes has been described by Silberberg and Gerritsen.[104] In this animal model they showed that the incidence of spondylosis was significantly elevated in the diabetic group relative to age-matched controls. The spondylotic changes observed in discs of these animals were comparable to those noted in degenerate human spines and included hyalinization and osteophyte formation at vertebral margins (see Chapter 12 for a detailed discussion of the pathology of spondylosis). In addition to the vertebral changes, disc prolapse occurred more frequently in the diabetic hamsters than in the control group. Significantly, however, tissue and cellular abnormalities were seen in both normal and spondylitic discs of the diabetic group which could not be attributed to mechanical attrition or the aging process. From these observations it was concluded that a systemic factor could be responsible. Since anterior pituitary growth hor- mones had previously produced effects in cartilage and vertebral bone[105-107] similar to the abnormalities found in the discs of the diabetic hamsters, it was suggested that these changes were attributable to hormones.

In a preliminary study of the intervertebral discs from four diabetic and two nondiabetic cadavers,[108] significant biochemical changes were noted in discs of the diabetic group. These results are summarized in Table 3. As is evident, the collagen content of the NP of discs from the diabetic group was found to be higher than the levels in the control discs. On the other hand, total hexosamine, which may be considered as an index of PG content, was substantially lower. Lysosomal enzymes involved in the intracellular processing of glycos- aminoglycans were also elevated, as was uridine diphosphate glucose dehydrogenase (UDPGDH), which is a marker enzyme for carbohydrate biosynthesis (Table 4). These important findings provide clear evidence of premature degenerative changes in the NP of discs of diabetic subjects. As PGs are lost from these tissues while collagen content is increased, a decline in disc resilience and swelling pressure would be anticipated to result in abnormal mechanical stresses on both disc tissues and vertebrae. Therefore, spondylotic changes in the spine of diabetics would seem to be influenced by systemic factors. It is to be expected that with the passage of time and additional research the hormone or hormones implicated will be identified. Such data would be of immense value in providing some insight into the role that hormones may play in the turnover of normal discs tissues as well as growth and aging disturbances (e.g., senility).

IV. CHEMONUCLEOLYSIS

The concept of introducing a specific enzyme into a degenerate disc to bring about a transformation to a more dense connective tissue was first noted by Carl Hirsch in 1959.[109] The suggestion was based on his many years of study on the spine in which he observed that back pain arising from instability and rupture of the AF was essentially eliminated when

Table 3

RESULTS OF THE BIOCHEMICAL COMPOSITION OF THE
INTERVERTEBRAL DISCS OF DIABETIC AND NONDIABETIC PATIENTS
(MEAN ± SE)

	Annulus		Nucleus	
	Control (5)	Diabetic (15)	Control (5)	Diabetic (15)
Total collagen/hydroxyproline, mg/g d.w.	67.4 ± 7.9	67.7 ± 3.8	49.0 ± 7.2	64.6 ± 2.9[a]
Acid-soluble collagen/hydroxyproline, μg/g d.w.	143.6 ± 14.3	207.3 ± 22.3	507.6 ± 68.6	170.3 ± 40.6[a]
Hexosamine, mg/g d.w.	402 ± 34	378 ± 45	542 ± 59	366 ± 42[a]
Hexuronic acid, mg/g d.w.	478 ± 42	409 ± 39	579 ± 55	456 ± 33
Calcium, mg/g d.w.	35.3 ± 7.8	42.8 ± 4.1	34.1 ± 3.7	42.1 ± 2.3
Magnesium, mg/g d.w.	4.80 ± 0.67	5.31 ± 0.30	5.36 ± 0.30	6.65 ± 0.56
Inorganic phosphorus, mg/g d.w.	1.07 ± 0.16	0.89 ± 0.11	0.90 ± 0.21	1.16 ± 0.27
Citrate, mg/g d.w.	2.19 ± 0.79	3.08 ± 0.68	2.86 ± 0.78	3.70 ± 0.65

Note: Number of samples is indicated in parentheses. SE, standard error; d.w., dry weight.

[a] $p < 0.05$.

From Aufdermaur et al., *Exp. Cell Biol.*, 48, 89, 1980. With permission.

Table 4

ENZYME ACTIVITIES IN INTERVERTEBRAL DISCS OF DIABETIC AND
NONDIABETIC SUBJECTS (MEAN ± SE)

	Annulus		Nucleus	
	Control (5)	Diabetic (15)	Control (5)	Diabetic (15)
β-Glucuronidase, μM/kg d.w./hr	67 ± 22	88 ± 31	45 ± 12	180 ± 43[a]
β-Acetyl galactosaminidase, μM/kg d.w./hr	246 ± 49	230 ± 51	173 ± 35	415 ± 57[a]
β-Acetylglucosaminidase, μM/kg d.w./hr	3.67 ± 1.06	2.91 ± 0.56	1.91 ± 0.35	5.24 ± 0.95[b]
UDPGDH, mM/kg d.w./hr	3.21 ± 1.70	6.27 ± 1.47	2.84 ± 0.80	11.48 ± 2.42[a]
PFK, μM/kg d.w./hr	754 ± 199	394 ± 31	609 ± 76	572 ± 129
Noncollagen protein, g/kg d.w.	45.4 ± 6.5	29.9 ± 4.1	50.3 ± 4.6	39.4 ± 4.3
DNA, mg/g d.w.	0.46 ± 0.17	0.67 ± 0.24	0.52 ± 0.10	0.46 ± 0.07

Note: Number of samples is indicated in parentheses. SE, standard error; d.w., dry weight.

[a] $p < 0.01$.
[b] $p < 0.001$.

From Aufdermaur et al., *Exp. Cell Biol.*, 48, 89, 1980, S. Karger AG, Basel. With permission.

a degenerate disc was transformed, as occurs with trauma and aging, into a dense, less mobile tissue. Such an inelastic structure was postulated to be less capable of distortion under mechanical loading and thus would exert minimal stress on nerve fibers on the periphery of the annulus and longitudinal ligament. These were considered to be the source of the back pain. The use of a chondrolytic enzyme which, when introduced into the disc, would accelerate the degenerative process, was proposed. While this suggestion was based on an oversimplification of a multifactoral problem that is addressed in some detail in Chapters 5 (Volume 1) and 11, it did provide the stimulus for a biochemical approach to the treatment of disorders of the intervertebral disc. A chondrolytic enzyme was found by Lyman Smith in 1964,[110] and today chemonucleolysis is well established but not universally accepted as an alternative to traditional surgical techniques.

A variety of enzyme preparations have been used as nucleolytic agents. The list includes collagenase, hyaluronidase, trypsin, chymotrypsin, papain, and chymopapain. However, chymopapain is by far the most widely investigated preparation and has spawned an extensive and highly controversial literature.

The present review does not attempt to provide an exhaustive coverage on chemonucleolysis, but rather to highlight publications which have contributed to our overall understanding of these agents, particularly with regard to their mechanism of action, clinical efficacy, and toxicity.

A. Chymopapain

On the basis of early studies by Thomas,[111] who demonstrated that rabbit elastic and hyaline cartilage could be degraded in vivo by the intravenous administration of crude papain, Smith et al.[110,112] proposed the use of this or similar enzymes to depolymerize the noncollaginous components of the NP of the disc. Since, it was realized that the papain preparation originally used by Thomas[111] was crude and contained other enzymes, such as chymopapain and lysozyme, each of these was individually tested for chondrolytic properties using young rabbits. Papain and chymopapain, but not lysozyme, were found to be very effective in degrading the proteoglycan-rich NP of the rabbits used. Moreover, it did so in a concentration-dependent manner, as was shown radiographically by loss of disc height and by the dissolution of the NP when viewed at autopsy. When these enzymes were administered at high doses or intrathecally, hemorrhage and breakdown of paraspinal tissues were demonstrated. Similar findings were subsequently reported by others.[113-115] Chymopapain was eventually selected for more detailed investigation because of its narrow specificity and lower toxicity compared to papain.

B. Experimental Studies with Chymopapain

Chymopapain is a cysteine proteinase (E.C. 3.4.22.6) which may be extracted with papain and lysozyme from papaya latex.[116] It is a proteinase with a broad specificity of action, which nevertheless is narrower than that of papain. It will hydrolyze most proteins at neutral to alkaline pHs and, like other cysteine proteinases, requires activation by disulfide reduction or by thiol exchange agents such as cysteine or mercaptoethanol for optimum activity. In its reduced (sulfydryl) form it is susceptible to inactivation by heavy metals. For this reason, metal chelators such as disodium EDTA are usually added to chymopapain preparations to maintain activity. The use of chymopapain as a chemonucleolytic agent depends on its ability to cleave the protein core of PGs present in the NP. The glycosaminoglycans (with polypeptide stubs attached) released by this hydrolysis may be further metabolized to oligosaccharides by disc cells or diffuse out of the disc via the capillaries on the periphery of the AF or through the cartilaginous end-plate (see Chapter 9). That such a process does take place in vivo was demonstrated by the finding of increased levels of glycosaminoglycans in the sera and urine of patients undergoing intradiscal chymopapain treatment.[27,117]

An essential requirement for the successful application of chymopapain as a chemonucleolytic agent is that the concentration used for dissolution of NP PGs does not cause damage to the AF or cartilaginous end-plate. While the major structural components of the AF are type I and II collagens (see Volume 1, Chapter 7), which in their native state are reported to be inert to chymopapain,[118,119] this tissue also contains PGs, which would be readily degraded by this enzyme. Moreover, the cartilaginous end-plates, which are hyaline cartilage and thus contain a high proportion of PGs, would also be susceptible to chymopapain. Thus, chymopapain does not show a particular specificity for the NP of the disc. However, the extent of degradation which eventually occurs would be highly dependent on the activity of the enzyme preparation used and the amount injected. Furthermore, strong binding of this enzyme to substrate molecules has been shown to occur,[111,120] and, provided the binding sites in the NP do not become saturated, the sphere of proteolytic activity would be confined to this tissue. Rabbits and mongrel dogs were used in the early experiments to assess the tissue specificity of chymopapain as a function of dosage.[112,113] These studies showed that injections as low as 0.08 mg per disc of the enzyme were effective in selectively depolymerizing the PGs of the NP.

Subsequent investigations[119,121] using immature beagles provided the first evidence that reconstitution of the NP could take place following intradiscal chymopapain administration. Nuclear dissolution was observed within 7 to 9 days of administration of 0.1 mg of the then commercially available chymopapain preparation known as Discase®.[119,121] This preparation also contained cysteine and disodium EDTA as enzyme activators. The extent of recovery of disc height was determined radiographically after 3, 6, 9, 12, 15, 18, 20, 22, and 24 months. While almost complete recovery in disc height in these animals was achieved 2 years after administration of the low-dose (0.1 mg) Discase®, this was found not to occur when higher concentrations (1.0 to 10 mg) were used. Microscopic examination of disc tissues at post-mortem 1 month after injection of high-dose chymopapain revealed damage to the cartilaginous end-plate and vertebral bodies. However, the AF remained free of such lesions. From this important study Garvin and Jennings[121] concluded that the extent of regeneration of the NP was related to the viability of the chondrocytes remaining in the tissue after chymopapain treatment. They acknowledged that the animals used in their experiments were young and noted that the regrowth phenomena in the few older beagles studied was more variable.

A subsequent study[122] confirmed these observations but also demonstrated the release into the bloodstream of immulogically detectable fragments of chymopapain after its use in both dogs and humans. In view of the rapid inactivation of chymopapain by serum α-2-macroglobulin, these fragments, if active, were unlikely to cause systemic damage.

The matter remained dormant for nearly 20 years until reopened by Bradford et al. in 1983.[123,124] In contrast to the earlier studies, the constitution of the regrown NP was examined both histologically and biochemically. Six months after its dissolution in dogs the reconstituted NP was found to contain PGs of composition similar to those extracted from untreated discs. The biomechanical properties of the reconstituted discs were also examined and showed characteristics comparable to controls. Unfortunately the number of animals used in this study was extremely small, and their ages and breed types were unknown. This is a particularly important point since, as noted earlier by Garvin and Jennings,[121] older dogs were known to respond to chemonucleolysis less favorably than younger animals, which would be expected to have more viable disc cells.[132] Furthermore, the NP of the discs of mature chondrodystrophoid breeds (e.g., the beagle, dachshund, and basset hound[125,126]) have a much higher collagen and lower PG content than the nonchondrodystrophoid breeds (e.g., the greyhound[127-130]). The response of the chondrodystrophoid NP to chymopapain treatment could, for these reasons alone, be expected to be different to discs of the nonchondrodystrophoid breeds.

A recent comparative study[131] of the effects of chymopapain chemonucleolysis and surgical excision of NP (discectomy) on the mechanical properties of the canine intervertebral disc revealed little difference in the outcome of these two procedures. Adult beagles were used, and discs examined 6 weeks and 5 months after either treatment. The relative stiffness values, including axial compression, anterior-posterior bending, and lateral-medial bending, were measured for intact spines; the chymopapain group showed a 50% loss in torsional stiffness and a decline in bending stiffness 6 weeks postoperatively. After 5 months both treatment groups demonstrated increased medial-lateral bending stiffness. At autopsy, 5 months after surgery, the discectomy group showed the presence of fibrocartilage replacement in the surgically created defects. Surprisingly, however, the NP of the chymopapain-treated groups appeared normal with regard to saffranin-*O* staining and cellular appearance 6 weeks and 5 months postinjection. As other workers,[123,124] as well as our own unpublished studies, have demonstrated, only marginal reconstitution of the NP occurs in periods of less than 3 months. It is likely that the levels of active chymopapain achieved in the discs in the above study were only sufficient to achieve partial dissolution of the NP proteoglycans.

C. Toxicity and Side Effects of Chymopapain

The local and systemic toxic effects of chymopapain have been studied using rabbits,[112,113,115,119] dogs,[113,121,133] cats,[134,135] and hamsters.[115] In some cases results by one group have not been reproduced by others using the same concentrations of enzyme as determined on a basis of mass. This discrepency probably arises from the wide variation in true enzyme activity in different commercial preparations of chymopapain coupled with its relatively low stability in solution at room temperature. In principal, all experimental studies should be undertaken using freshly prepared solutions of a purified preparation of the enzyme, the activity of which has been assessed in terms of an internationally acceptable unit. The description of an experimental finding as resulting from a particular concentration of chymopapain is of no real value unless the enzyme activity of unit mass of the preparation used is known. Such enzyme activity units are easily determined by monitoring the rate of degradation of a synthetic substrate (usually *N*-benzoyl-DL-arginine-*p*-nitroanilide) by chymopapain under a predetermined set of experimental conditions (time, temperature, enzyme concentration, substrate concentration, and buffer pH). The problem may be further compounded by the known instability of chymopapain in solution due to aerial oxidation and inactivation by heavy metals. Commercial preparations may vary in their stability due to the types of antioxidants included or the presence of impurities, such as heavy metals, which could modify biological activity of the activated form. For example, the two chymopapain preparations approved for chemonucleolysis in the U.S. — Chymodiactin® (Smith Laboratories) and Discase® (Baxter-Travenol Laboratories) — when examined for stability in solution under identical conditions showed the former preparation to be much more stable over 24 hr than the latter.[136] This result is shown in Figure 6. Such experiments clearly demonstrate the need to undertake steps to standardize the preparations to be used for both laboratory and clinical investigations.

Notwithstanding the above comments, some important observations have been made on the toxicological effects of chymopapain. Dogs administered intradiscally more than 180 mg of chymopapain succumbed within 24 hr.[132] Autopsy showed extensive hemorrhage in vital organs, including the kidneys, lungs, gastrointestinal tract, abdominal cavities, and thorax. Since hemorrhage also occurred in paravertebral muscles as well as in epidural and intrathecal tissues adjacent to the injection sites, it is likely that, at the concentration used, chymopapain eventually leaked from the discs and entered the bloodstream. At this high dosage level, the inhibitory capacity of α-2-macroglobulin and other proteinase inhibitors would be exceeded.

The severe toxicity associated with the peri- and intradural localization of low-dosage chymopapain was demonstrated by Widdowson[133] using 62 adult dogs. In some cases paraplegia was generally produced, accompanied by spinal cord demyelination, and vascular and inflammatory reactions around the dura. The pathological manifestations were even more severe when the enzyme was injected into the subarachnoid space or spinal cord. These findings were in agreement with those of Shealy,[134] who used cats and noted that hemorrhage,

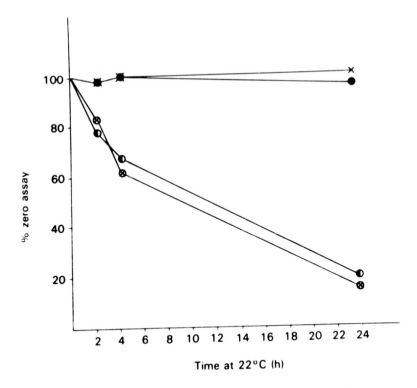

FIGURE 6.   The effect of storage on reconstituted chymopapain from two different sources. Two batches of Chymodiactin®, BM201 (●) and BM 301 (×), and two batches of Discase®, AV158B (⊗) and AV15F8D (◐), were examined. Activity was determined using BAPNA as substrate at 2, 4, and 24 hr after reconstitution. Results were expressed as the percentage of activity measured at zero time. As can be seen, once reconstituted, Discase® is less stable with time than Chymodiactin®. (From Cockayne, D. et al., *Current Concepts in Chemonucleolysis*, Sutton, J. C., Ed., Royal Society of Medicine, International Congress Symposium Series, 1985. With permission.)

major vascular changes, cell necrosis, and inflammation were prominent features of injecting the chymopapain into the epidural space, cerebral cortex, subarachnoid space, and carotid adventitia. Similar experiments by Ford,[135] however, failed to demonstrate the severe toxic effects of this enzyme after extradural administration.

The intrathecal toxicity of chymopapain was again highlighted by the studies of Garvin et al.[113] and Gesler,[114] where death in dogs was produced by this route of administration. The effects of chymopapain on the peripheral vascular bed in the hamster cheek pouch, rabbit ear, and rabbit tibial nerves was investigated by Branemark et al.[115] using a well-defined Discase® preparation. This group showed that the microcirculation in these tissues was damaged by chymopapain in a dose-dependent manner accompanied by disruption of the endothelium and vascular walls. While the rabbit tibial nerves were more resistant to damage than the vascular beds, the spectrum of pathological changes observed was similar. Electron microscopy studies also showed that endothelial cells and blood corpuscles were injured after exposure of the rabbit mesentery to chymopapain. A recent study by Zook and Kobrine[137] using cynomolgus monkeys supports the conclusion of Branemark et al.[115]

For the most part, the toxicological studies described above can be attributed to the proteolytic attack by chymopapain on glycoproteins and PGs which are structural components of the extracellular matrix of these tissues. Blood vessels walls, lung and kidney basement membranes, and outher sheath nerve tissues all contain types III, IV, and V collagen in varying proportions as the major structural proteins.[138] Since the toxicological studies showed that such connective tissues were susceptible to degradation by chymopapain, it would appear that the collagen types cited may, unlike the type I and II collagens of cartilage and the intervertebral disc, be susceptible to attack by chymopapain. While this question remains to be answered experimentally, it is noteworthy that type II, IV, and V collagens can be cleaved by broad specificity proteinase such as granulocyte elastase, trypsin, and certain cathepsins.[139]

Examined in this light, chymopapain could be considered as a therapeutic agent with inherent problems. While this may be so, it should be borne in mind that when used correctly its sphere of influence should be confined to the intervertebral disc, where it binds strongly to its substrate molecules, which are usually in excess. Even so, it has been estimated by Wiltse et al.[140,141] that some leakage of enzyme into the epidural space does occur in about 25% of discs injected with chymopapain. Provided the amounts released are small, damage is probably minimal.

However, major mishaps have occurred, generally through errors of needle placement, and chymopapain has been released into the spinal canal or upon peridiscal structures. Under such conditions, chymopapain may enter the bloodstream, producing anaphylaxis. In evaluating 2000 patients treated with chymopapain in 1980, McCulloch[142] estimated that the frequency of anaphylaxis was 0.6%. A study by Smith Laboratories in 1984 of 28,924 patients who had been given the chymopapain preparation Chymodiactin indicated an anaphylaxis incidence of 0.7%. Of interest was the finding that the frequency was much higher in females (1.2%) than males (0.4%). Several deaths from anaphylaxis have been recorded,[143,144] and the fatality rate has now recently been estimated as 0.15%.[145] Some individuals are sensitized to chymopapain, possibly due to ingestion of the antigen from other sources, e.g., consumption of papaya or meat tenderizers.

It is now recommended that prospective patients be screened for chymopapain allergy prior to chemonucleolysis. Preoperative chymopapain sensitivity tests have been described[145-147] which can detect and quantitate the presence of chymopapain antibodies in patient sera. As a further precaution, it is recommended that users of chymopapain maintain, close at hand, resuscitative and other measures (epinephrine, cortisone, and fluid substitutes) for treating anaphylactic shock.

Other recorded complications arising from the use of chymopapain include paraplegia[143,148] and discitis.[149,150] The incidence of the latter is reported as 22 cases in a group of 29,075 patients and may be attributable to inadequate sterile techniques. However, the possible presence of microorganisms in faulty commercial chymopapain preparations cannot be totally excluded.

D. Clinical Studies with Chymopapain

In 1964, Smith, encouraged by experimental studies achieved by intradiscal administration of chymopapain in rabbits[112] and paraplegic dogs,[151] initiated the first clinical trial with this enzyme.[152] Ten patients were selected on the basis of their incapacitating sciatica and the fact that they normally would have been candidates for surgery. Each was administered a different amount of chymopapain, generally in two discs, one or both having been judged to be abnormal. Within 24 hr seven of the ten patients were free of sciatic and back pain. One of the remaining nonresponders had a sequestered fragment at the L5 nerve root, and the two remaining patients showed some recovery from pain with time. The number of patients treated by this technique was enlarged to 75 by 1965,[152] and by 1972 it was reported[153] that more than 20 investigators had given 15,000 patients chymopapain. However, from that period up to 1974, no group had undertaken a truly randomized double-blind drug trial employing this method of treatment.

A contributory factor to the reluctance by early workers to undertake a double-blind trial was the need to inject saline, or the chymopapain vehicle, into symptomatic discs. Such a procedure was anticipated to increase the patients' pain and could have medicolegal consequences. Because of this, numerous clinical studies, mainly in the U.S. and Canada,[140,154-175] consisted of open trials with small patient numbers and short-term follow-up periods. Patients were generally selected for treatment according to Smith's original criteria, and success was measured in terms of the reduction of pain and the return to normal activity. Thus, results were considered excellent if the patient was completely asymptomatic within a few months of treatment but only fair if pain and/or discomfort was intermittent and they were required to undertake lighter work. Failure, described as a poor result, occurred when back surgery was required to eliminate the pain. For the most part these early trials demonstrated, using the criteria described, the overall effectiveness of intradiscal chymopapain for the treatment of sciatic pain. Failures were generally associated with sequestration of disc material or incorrect diagnoses for the cause of the back pain in the first place, e.g., spondylosis. A detailed analysis of these early clinical trials is described by Simmons et al.[176]

During this period, chymopapain was vigorously opposed by many surgeons, and its therapeutic value compared to its placebo effect was much debated. Several reviews[176-181] make interesting reading and describe an almost month-by-month account of the tumultuous events leading up to the withdrawal of chymopapain as Discase® by Baxter-Travenol in 1975. This action was taken on the recommendation of the U.S. Food and Drug Administration (FDA), which thought that a classical randomized double-blind trial was then the only reasonable way to resolve the contentious issue surrounding the use of this drug.

The first U.S.-based double-blind trials with chymopapain were undertaken between 1974 and 1975 by Brown and Daroff,[182] Schwetschenau et al.,[183] Martins et al.,[153] and Javid et al.[184] One hundred and five patients were reported to have participated; however, details of only 66 were reported fully. The chymopapain-treated group received 1.0 mℓ (2.5 nanakatal* units) of the enzyme provided by Baxter-Travenol Laboratories in the form of Discase®. The control group was injected intradiscally with a 1.0-mℓ solution containing the enzyme activator cysteine hydrochloride, disodium EDTA, and the X-ray contrast medium sodium isothalamate. A criteria of success or failure was whether the trial drug code was requested to be broken by the patient and/or investigator. If this occurred the solution administered initially was considered to be a failure. The outcome of these trials, after a short-term (6-month) and a long-term (12-month) follow-up period, showed no statistically significant difference between the enzyme-treated and the control groups. These findings were not well received, for they contrasted with the many previous nonrandomized series (previously cited) as well as with open trials[185-187] of chymopapain treatment vs. surgery. An explanation offered for the failure of the double-blind study was that the dosage of chymopapain used was too low since 2 mℓ (5.0 kat units) per disc was the dosage normally[188] recommended by the manufacturer. It was also suggested that the principal investigators participating in the trial lacked experience in the techniques of chemonucleolysis as well as in the proper selection of patients for such a study. Finally, it was argued that the materials used in the control group (i.e., cysteine and EDTA) could have had a therapeutic effect themselves and thus did not constitute a true placebo.

Although the in vivo effectiveness of the cysteine-EDTA combination was not established, it was recommended by the FDA that all subsequent clinical trials use sterile saline as the control preparation. Accordingly, a double-blind trial of chymopapain against saline placebo was undertaken.[189,190] In this study 60 patients with strictly defined unilateral sciatic pain originating from nerve root involvement and a posterolateral disc herniation were selected. Moreover, the patients participating in the trial had failed to respond to traditional conserv-

---

* One nanakatal unit of chymopapain activity would liberate 1 nmol of *p*-nitroaniline per second from *N*-α-benzoyl-DL-argenine-*p*-nitroanilide substrate at pH 6.4 and 37°C.

ative management for 6 months before commencing the trial and would normally have been candidates for surgery. The group was randomly divided into two groups of equal size. One group received 2 mℓ sterile saline intradiscally and the other group 2 mℓ (8 mg) chymopapain as Discase®, both placebo and drug being administered by a blind procedure. Patients were interviewed at 6 weeks, 3 months, and 2 years after intradiscal treatment, and in no instance was the drug code broken. The follow-up examination included both patient and investigator assessment of results as determined by pain relief. Failures were treated by laminectomy. The results of this study showed a statistically significant difference between the chymopapain-treated and saline-treated groups. Patient self-assessment showed that the placebo group improved from 37% to 57% over the first 6 months, whereas the chymopapain recipients showed improvement from 73% to 80% over the same period. Investigator assessment at 6 months indicated a response similar to patient self-assessment. Additional assessments 2 years[190] after initial chymopapain treatment demonstrated that the 6-month findings were sustained, leading to the conclusion that relative to saline, for a carefully selected group of patients, chymopapain may have a real therapeutic role.

Chymodiactin® was used in a double-blind trial against saline placebo at seven centers in the U.S. in 1981.[191] Again, patients were carefully selected to comply with the criteria of persistent radicular pain and neurological defects that did not respond to 6 weeks of conservative therapy. One hundred and eight patients participated and were followed for up to 6 months. Placebo failures were, unlike the situation in the Australian study,[189,190] allowed Chymodiactin® treatment within 6 weeks of failure, a practice which constituted a code break protocol. An 82% success rate relative to 41% placebo success rate was reported, using both patients and investigator means of assessment.

These recent double-blind clinical trials appear to have eliminated the argument concerning the placebo effect of chemonucleolysis. Others have challenged the advantage of chymopapain over surgery.[192,193] Furthermore, there is as yet no data which compare well-defined, long-term, conservative measures against intradiscal chymopapain.[194] The estimated long-term success rate for conservative therapy[198] in which compliance has been observed was 75%, which was the same as a 12-year follow-up of a chymopapain-treated group by Parkinson.[171]

E. Use of Chemonucleolysis in Adolescents

Disc prolapse is not common in children or adolescents, but for those who appear resistant to conservative measures surgical methods are generally employed when symptoms demand. The possible use of chemonucleolysis for the treatment of disc prolapse in children was discussed by Watts in 1983.[196] On the basis that the juvenile disc contains a higher proportion of degradable PGs than the corresponding aged tissue, he argued that the subsequent loss of disc height which would occur following chemonucleolysis could lead to biomechanical alterations in the spine resulting in potential problems in later years.

Dunlop and Hutton,[195] using cadaveric lumbar spines within the age range of 31 to 70 years, demonstrated that a decrease in disc height of 1 to 4 mm produced by compression in a hydraulic press caused a marked increase ($\geq$33%) in peak pressures across the facet joints. This order of disc narrowing invariably occurs after chemonucleolysis and suggests that osteoarthrotic changes may arise in these joints with time. Of course, this situation may not eventuate if reconstitution of the NP takes place. This is reported[201] to occur occasionally in adults, but no sound data are available describing the frequency of the recovery in disc height.

Since disc viability and metabolic activity are high in the younger age groups,[132] it is reasonable to expect that NP reconstitution would occur more readily in the adolescent. As already indicated, experiments in young dogs[119,121,123,124] support such a hypothesis when appropriate levels of chymopapain have been administered.[121] At high concentrations of this enzyme not only were the components of the extracellular matrix degraded, but disc cell viability was undoubtedly compromised, presumably due to enzymatic damage to cell membrane proteins. A recent report[197] using 55 patients aged between 13 and 19 years with symptoms and myelographic evidence of disc prolapse at one or two lower lumbar levels provides no detail of the amounts of chymopapain administered. While a 49% success rate was found 8 weeks posttreatment, 80% of the group was considered to be asymptomatic in the long-term follow-up period of 2 to 12 years (4.5 years average). As these data were collected by means of questionnaires and telephone interviews, no assessment could be made of the long-term status of the chymopapain-treated discs. Such information would have been of considerable value in the debate concerning the reconstitution of the NP in man as a function of age.

At the time of this writing, 12 adolescents with proven lumbar disc prolapse are under treatment in the Department of Orthopaedic and Traumatic Surgery at The Royal North Shore Hospital of Sydney. Each patient received a single-level injection of chymopapain using a standard technique. So far all the patients have had a satisfactory clinical response with symptoms abating at a variable rate over 6 weeks postinjection. On the other hand, the clinical tension signs, which are invariably marked in adolescent disc prolapse, subsided more slowly, and at a rate comparable to that seen after simple disectomy. Of the radiographs taken at 6 weeks postinjection, a 25 to 50% decrease in disc height was demonstrated, and in adolescent disc prolapse this is usually near normal. Six of these patients have been followed for more than 12 months, and none as yet has radiographic evidence of disc reconstitution.

F. Mechanism of Action of Chymopapain

As previously indicated, it has been demonstrated both in vitro and in vivo that chymopapain can rapidly depolymerize the PGs and glycoproteins of the NP. Since these macromolecules confer to disc tissues the properties of water retention and turgidity, their depletion from the extracellular matrix would rapidly lead to a decrease in disc height. Whether the loss in disc height and/or other intradiscal changes induced by chymopapain injection are responsible for the observed pain relief and amelioration of neurological signs is not presently known. The answer to this question is obviously of some importance, particularly as studies have shown that 60 to 70% of back pain sufferers show spontaneous resolution of symptoms using conservative measures.[198]

Anatomical studies to show that the periphery of the intervertebral disc does possess a nerve supply have been described in Chapter 5 (Volume 1). In addition, the anterior and longitudinal ligaments which are in direct contact with, and physically support, the annulus are also innervated. The intervertebral disc and associated ligaments are thus potential sources of pain, which, as has been discussed in Chapter 5, can be provoked by distention of the AF during intradiscal injection of saline or X-ray contrast media.

Degenerative changes in the AF of the disc with aging, which are frequently seen in autopsy specimens as annular fissures and rents extending centripedally, posteriorly, or in a posterolateral direction (see Chapter 11), could, because of the inherent weakness they introduce to this structure, lead to its bulging under axial loading. This distention of the intact AF beyond its normal confines may, on the basis of the above, produce pain sensations similar to those obtained by the intradiscal administration of fluids. However, such stress acting on nerve endings or nerve roots sensitized by inflammatory mediators would result in heightened and more sustained pain perception (for a discussion of this point, see Green[66]).

In his publication on the mechanism of action of chymopapain in ruptured lumbar disc disease, Watts[199] draws our attention to the selectivity of pain production which can be achieved by stimulating nerve fibers in different regions of the longitudinal ligament and annulus. Applying the studies of Murphy,[20,200] he points out that physical stimulation of the midline region of the posterior longitudinal ligament produced back pain in patients undergoing operation for lumbar disc rupture. However, stimulation of lateral regions of this ligament or the posterolateral aspects of the annulus induced both back pain and radial leg pain typical of nerve root compression. Stimulation of these nerve endings can thus reproduce some of the clinical symptoms of sciatica without resorting to the clinical explanation of nerve root entrapment or irritation. Internal decompression of the disc by chemonucleolysis could thus reduce tensional stresses on the AF and longitudinal ligaments, thereby providing symptomatic relief. In this context, it is important to note that nerve root irritation produced by disc fragment sequestration could not be expected to respond to chemonucleolysis, and indeed many of the clinical failures to this procedure have, at the time of surgery, demonstrated the presence of disc fragments in the spinal canal.

Watts[199] also proposes an additional explanation for the mode of action of chymopapain which is independent of the "internal decompression theory" described above. This theory is based on the common clinical observation that degenerate discs injected with contrast media frequently demonstrate radiographically the flow of contrast media along fissures in the annulus. These annular tears or channels often extended to the outer AF regions, which, as already described, are endowed with nerve endings. It is assumed that the chymopapain solution, when introduced into the NP of a degenerate disc would, like the X-ray contrast media, migrate along the fissures, eventually perfusing those regions of the AF which contain sensory fibers. It is proposed that these would then be attacked by the enzyme to produce a total or partial neurectomy. In support of the direct action of chymopapain on nerve fibers was the clinical observation of Watts[199] and others[201-203] that some individuals show almost instantaneous relief (1 to 2 hr) of pain following chemonucleolysis. However, as enzymes generally take some time to degrade their substrates and disc height has not been reported to alter significantly within a few hours after chymopapain injection, the possibility exists that these claims may be due to a placebo effect.

A more serious criticism of the concept of chymopapain neurectomy is whether this enzyme, at the concentrations used clinically, is capable of degrading the protective sheaves of nerve tissues. As already discussed, chymopapain, while a broad-specificity proteinase, is reported to be incapable of degrading native types I and II collagen. On the other hand, the loose connective tissue, including the epineural and perineural sheaves of peripheryl nerves, contains several other collagen types (III, IV, and V) apart from type I, which may be more susceptible to degradation by chymopapain. Certainly, at high concentrations, chymopapain has been demonstrated to produce damage to peripheral nerves[115,137,204] and subdural tissues (as cited above) in several species, lending some experimental support to the chymopapain neurectomy theory.

G. Collagenase

After chymopapain, collagenase ranks as the most extensively investigated chemonucleolytic agent. Its use in this area was initially suggested by Sussman[205,206] on the premise that collagen represented a much larger proportion of the extracellular matrix of a degenerate NP than PGs, and therefore a more rational approach for its dissolution would be to use an enzyme with specificity for this protein. The collagenase preparation proposed for this purpose was that derived from cultures of *Clostridium histolyticum*, and since it was known that this bacterium also produces a variety of other enzymes with elastase-like, trypsin-like, and pepidase activities, extensive purification was necessary prior to its application.

Using such preparations it was demonstrated that the NP and part of the AF of dog and monkey discs as well as human disc tissue obtained at surgery could be readily degraded.[207,208] In these early experiments a wide margin of safety was indicated between the concentration of enzyme effective for degradation of the disc NP and that which would also cause damage to extradural and paraspinal tissues. Intrathecal administration did, however, produce subarachnoid hemorrhage and degradation of surrounding collaginous structures. Using a crude preparation of *C. histolyticum* collagenase, Garvin[209] showed much more severe toxic effects when this preparation was administered to rabbits and mongrel dogs than reported by Sussman[207] and by Bromley et al.[208] Intradiscal injections at doses as low as 6 units per disc produced digestion of rabbit NP as well as that part of the AF and ventral ligament violated by the needle used to introduce the enzyme. With higher doses (1500 units) it was reported that areas of complete digestion of the NP, AF, longitudinal ligament, and cartilaginous endplate occurred, accompanied by extensive hemorrhaging from the vertebral bodies. Epidural and intrathecal toxicity was also evident in Garvin's dog experiments, leading this investigator to report: "The sequelae of collagenase action whether injected intravenously, epidurally, or intrathecally were characterised by severe local and/or systemic hemorrhage. The toxicity of collagenase seemed to be associated with dissolution of the collagenous network supporting the capillaries and vessels of the microcirculation."

Subsequent studies using primates[210] confirmed these earlier observations and demonstrated erosion at the vertebral margins within 3 weeks of intradiscal administration of collagenase. Osteophyte formation and sclerosis were also evident after 9.5 months, and vertebral body fusion occurred in some animals after 13.5 months. Two recent toxicological studies of the effects of collagenase in the form of Nucleolysin® (Advance Biofactures Corporation and Knoll Pharmaceuticals) on rabbit and cynomolgus monkey's peripheral nerve tissues have been described.[137,211] Using clinical or subclinical concentrations in acute experiments, transient swelling at the site of application as well as the production of edema in the epineurium was demonstrated. However, the permeability of the perineurium or the endoneurial microvascular bed was not affected by collagenase at the concentration used. These authors reported that collagenase produced less deleterious effects to nerve functionality than did chymopapain when used at clinically relevant concentrations.

The collagenase preparations used by Garvin[209] and by Stern and Coulson[210] were undoubtedly contaminated with other proteinases. (Further information on this point and analytical data on the various bacterial collagenase preparations are available.[212,213]) These contaminating bacterial proteinases are thought to enhance the degradative capacity of collagenase, possibly by removing other glycoproteins in the extracellular matrix which serve to protect the collagen fibrils from collagenase or by releasing the collagen chains by cleavage of the teleopeptide regions (compare granulocyte elastase). It is not surprising, therefore, that these workers should obtain results which were at variance with the studies of Sussman[206,207] as well as those of recent workers[137,211] who used the highly purified collagenase preparations.

In drawing attention to these discrepancies in experimental design, I am in no way attempting to diminish the dangers which may be associated with the use of collagenase as a chemonucleolytic agent, but only to highlight the difficulty of interpreting the literature on this subject when enzyme preparations of different purity are used. Irrespective of its purity, bacterial collagenase, unlike chymopapain, does not bind to disc matrix components, and it is reported to remain stable in solution for up to 14 days.[120] While such properties are useful to the experimentalist studying this enzyme, they are distinct disadvantages clinically, should the enzyme escape from the confines of the disc.

Despite these potential difficulties, three open[214-216] and one double-blind[217] clinical trials were undertaken up to 1984 for the use of intradiscal collagenase in the treatment of lumbar disc herniations. Patients were selected for these trials on the basis of myelographic evidence of disc protrusion at a single intervertebral space and being refractory to conservative therapy. Using saline as the control, which could on request be replaced by collagenase, and also the standard criteria for clinical assessment, a 78 to 80% success rate was claimed.

In 1984, workers[120,218] in West Berlin reported severe toxic side effects in treating patients with low back pain and sciatica using a purified preparation of collagenase supplied by Knoll AG. Eight of the eleven patients subjected to collagenase chemonucleolysis did not respond to the treatment or were worsened by the procedure. At operation, all showed evidence of softening of epidural tissue, destruction of the posterial vertebral ligament, and thinning of the dura. Curettage of the intervertebral space revealed destruction of the cartilaginous end-plate and vertebral bone accompanied by hemorrhaging. Light and scanning electron microscopy examination of the spinal tissues collected at the level of chemonucleolysis confirmed the macroscopic observations and also showed matrix depletion, cellular necrosis, and occasional pockets of cell proliferation in the cartilaginous end-plate.

The fact that the results obtained by the German workers were obtained with collagenase prepared outside the U.S. would again seem to reinforce the point already made that the potency of this enzyme may vary considerably with its origins and in particular by contamination by other bacterial proteinases. The complexity of the situation may be summed up by the words of Sussman, who, in a letter to the *Journal of Neurosurgery,*[219] remarked: "We have found that collagenase which is made so pure that trace proteinase contamination is almost eliminated loses its collagenolytic properties."

H. Infusion of Other Enzymes and Aprotinin into the Disc

A short paper in the Soviet literature[220] reports that the proteolytic enzymes trypsin and chemopsin, when injected into the intervertebral disc of dogs, produce sclerosis. Dissolution of the NP by chemopsin was claimed to be followed by a replacement structure consisting of fibrous connective tissue. Intradiscal trypsin was also used by Gol et al.[221] in a study of 49 cases of back and sciatic pain accompanied by sensory and myelographic evidence of disc protrusion. Trypsin (as Parenzyme) at concentrations of 5.0 to 7.5 mg/mℓ was found to produce considerable pain at the time of intradiscal injection, and its effects on disc dissolution were slow and inferior to hyaluronidase given by the same route. Moreover, hyaluronidase was reported to be nonirritant to thecal tissue as the dosage levels (100 to 300 units) examined. The small number of patients employed for this study, combined with the use of multiple injections, sometimes with cortisone, as well as the absence of suitable controls, renders assessment of the outcome of this trial impossible. However, an experimental study by Oegema et al.[222] showed that trypsin and chymotrypsin produced only marginal reduction in disc height when injected at 1.0 mg/mℓ into discs of mongrel dogs.

Other enzymes examined intradiscally by this group included clostripain, pronase (from *Streptomyces griseus),* and protease K (from *Tritirachim album).* While clostripain caused extensive degradation of the disc and cartilaginous end-plate (compare bacterial collagenase), reconstitution did occur, but the newly synthesized PGs were of the immature type, i.e., of large hydrodynamic size and low keratan sulfate content. Discs injected with 1.0 mg of protease K were also degraded, but this was accompanied by the formation of peripheral osteophytes on the anterior lips of vertebral bodies. In some instances complete bony bridges were seen 6 months after injection of this enzyme. The most promising preparation appeared to be pronase. In discs treated with this enzyme, dissolution, followed by recovery to 90 to 100% of original disc height, was observed after 6 months. The morphology of the reconstituted disc tissues looked normal, and there was no evidence of damage to the cartilaginous end-plate.

Biochemical studies on the PGs of the pronase-treated reconstituted NP showed that the percentage aggregation, hydrodynamic size, and chondroitin sulfate-keratan sulfate ratios were similar to those of control discs. From these studies, it was concluded that enzymes other than chymopapain or collagenase may be used as chemonucleolytic agents. By facilitating reconstitution of a disc matrix which was essentially indistinguishable from normal tissue, such agents may be superior to those presently used clinically.

Based on the rationale that the installation of pressure-reducing substances into the degenerate intervertebral disc would relieve pressure on irritated nerve roots, Kramer and Laturnus[223,224] proposed the use of aprotinin (Trasylol®) for the treatment of sciatica. This approach was also used by Lesoin et al.[225] for the treatment of cervical disc protrusions. Although aprotinin is a low-molecular-weight cationic proteinase inhibitor and would not, like chymopapain or collagenase, depolymerize components of the extracellular matrix, these authors suggest that such polypeptides would form strong complexes with glycosaminoglycans, thereby reducing the disc swelling pressure. Unless the glycosaminoglycan-aprotinin complex produced was insoluble and precipitated from the system (which is highly unlikely), the explanation offered by Kramer and co-workers[223,224] for the mechanism of action of aprotinin would seem ill founded. (See Chapter 9 for a detailed explanation of disc swelling pressure and the contribution made by free ions and charged polymers.)

As discussed in Chapter 8, the disc contains a host of proteinases capable of degrading the components of the extracellular matrix. Under normal circumstances, the effects of these enzymes are modulated by endogenous inhibitors. However, in the pathological state, as has been demonstrated in degenerate articular cartilage[226] and fibrocartilage,[227] the levels of the activated proteinase may exceed the inhibitory capacity of the tissue, and degradation of PGs could proceed. In contrast to the partially degraded PGs of articular cartilage which can freely diffuse into synovial fluid, PG fragments of the disc appear to remain *in situ* for much longer periods, probably because of the diffusion barriers imposed by the cartilaginous end-plate.[228,229] If the biosynthesis of disc PGs is proceeding at a normal or elevated rate, a net pool of charged PG fragments may thus accumulate in the disc, resulting in an increase in osmotic pressure. If this explanation is correct, then the installation into the NP of a proteinase inhibitor would be expected to effectively dampen the excess proteolytic activity, thereby decreasing the population of degraded proteoglycans accumulating in the disc tissues. Since our studies (see Volume I, Chapter 8) on the activated proteinase of the human disc, Discin, showed that this enzyme was inhibited by aprotinin,[230] it is possible that the beneficial clinical effects reported by Kramer et al.[223,224] occurred by such a mechanism.

V. EPILOGUE

From the literature which has been reviewed in this chapter, it could be concluded that there are relatively few therapeutic measures currently available which have been satisfactorily shown to modify the constitution of the intervertebral disc. Chemonucleolysis would represent the most widely used procedure, yet basic information on the mechanism(s) by which dissolution of disc PGs can lead to the biosynthesis of a new matrix still remains unresolved. Of paramount importance would be knowledge concerning the mechanisms controlling cell division and matrix production in the disc and how these processes are influenced by the introduction of exogenous enzymes into the system. Such data could promote the development of methodologies designed specifically to rejuvenate the disc matrix rather than to eliminate the symptoms of back pain, which is the present approach.

In Chapter 8, we discuss our recent studies on some of the enzyme systems present within disc tissues which are responsible for turnover of its matrix components. The situation is extremely complex, and a fine balance appears to exist between the activation and inhibition of these enzyme systems by specific disc proteins. Future drug therapy may use this knowledge. The introduction of such inhibitors into degenerate discs could shift the metabolic balance in favor of the replenishment of matrix PGs, thereby restoring more youthful biomechanical properties.

Some support for such an experimental approach has recently been obtained in our own laboratories.[231] In this study, a group of aged beagles, which are a chondrodystroid canine breed[125,126] with a strong disposition for disc prolapse,[126] were administered Arteparon® subcutaneously at 2.0 mg/kg twice weekly for 6 months. Arteparon® is a semisynthetic polysulfated glycosaminoglycan used in the treatment of osteoarthritis.[232] Two months prior to sacrifice, all animals were administered Na^{35}SO$_4$ to label their disc PGs isotopically. A control group of age-matched beagles was similarly treated with this isotope. Disc PGs were extracted with 4.0 *M* GuHCl, purified by density gradient ultracentrifugation, and then subjected to get filtration chromatography.

As can be seen from Figure 7, the level of PG aggregation, as demonstrated by the species eluting in the void volume of the column, was higher in both NP and AF of the Arteparon®-treated group. Moreover, the hydrodynamic size of the PG subunits which were included in the column was also larger in the drug-treated animals than in the controls. These results, coupled with other analytical data, indicated that the PGs of the Arteparon®-treated beagle discs were less degraded during the 2-month experimental radiolabeling period than those of the control discs. That is, a systemically administered drug had decreased the rate of PG turnover in the aged discs of these animals.

We proposed that Arteparon® achieved this by inhibiting the enzymes involved in the turnover of PGs in the disc. This explanation was based on the known potent inhibitory activity of Arteparon® against various neutral proteinases[233,234] and lysosomal hydrolases,[235] all of which have been shown to degrade proteoglycans extracellularly or intracellularly. Evidence that Arteparon®, which has a molecular weight of approximately 10,000 daltons and high negative charge, did indeed enter and localize within disc tissues to allow inhibition was provided by an earlier study in rabbits[235] and is demonstrated in Figure 8.

In clinical practice, however, patients do not present before disc degeneration becomes symptomatic, and in these instances the introduction of enzyme inhibitors, such as Arteparon®, into the disc may be too late to reverse the matrix damage that has already occurred. The eventual solution to this problem may lie in early diagnosis and detection of those individuals in the community with a predisposition to disc disorders. With the advent of monoclonal antibodies specific for various regions of the disc PGs,[237] this proposition is now well within our capabilities and offers some hope for the future.

VI. ACKNOWLEDGMENTS

The author gratefully acknowledges the assistance of Ms. Janet MacKenney for the typing of this manuscript, Dr. M. Smith for assistance in the retrieval of references, and Mrs. Nancy Wilson for proofreading this manuscript.

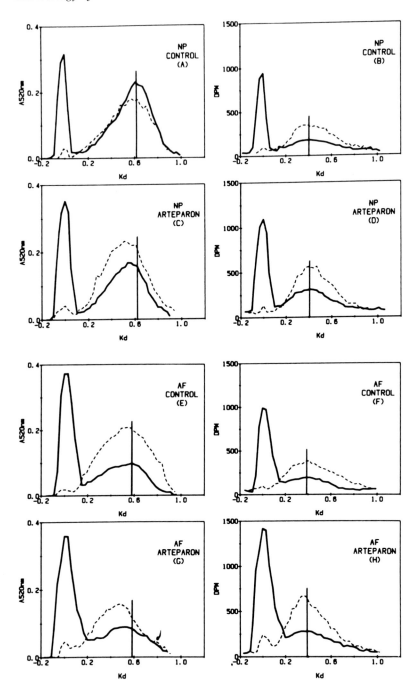

FIGURE 7.   The effect of Arteparon® on the hydrodynamic size and percentage aggregation of proteoglycans isolated from the beagle nucleus pulposus (NP) and annulus fibrosus (AF) is shown. Proteoglycan subunits were chromatographed on Sepharose CL 2B in the absence (---) and presence (———) of excess hyaluronate acid. Fractions were monitored for hexuronic acid (A520 nm) and radioactivity (DPM). As can be seen, the resident proteoglycan K_{av} of subunits isolated from discs of (C,G) Arteparon®-treated animals were smaller (K_{av} smaller) than (A,E) the nondrug-treated controls. This indicated that the hydrodynamic size of the proteoglycans in discs of drug-treated animals is larger than in the control. The proportion of proteoglycans which could aggregate in the presence of hyaluronic acid was also higher in the Arteparon®-treated group, as shown by the respective areas beneath the profiles of (A,G) the included fractions relative to (C,E) controls. (From Cole, T.-C., Ghosh P. and Taylor, T. K. F., unpublished.)

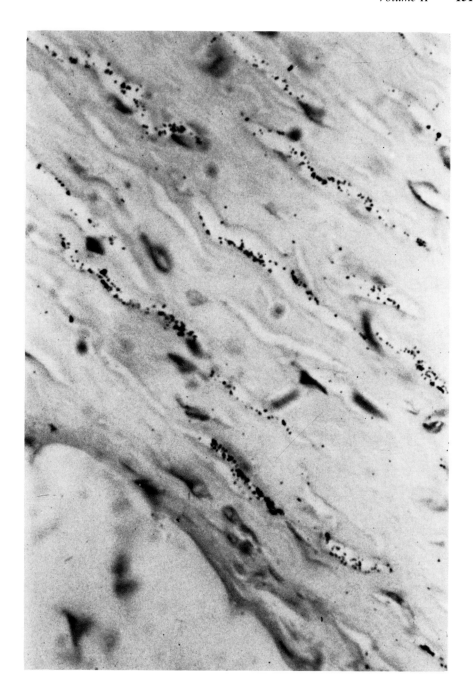

FIGURE 8.   Photomicroautograph of a horizontal hematoxylin-eosin-stained section of rabbit intervertebral disc showing the outer region of the annulus fibrosus 48 hr after intramuscular administration of ³H-Arteparon®. The radioactively labeled drug (visualized as silver grains) can be seen to be localized adjacent to collagen fibers, but this study[235] showed it was bound to a noncollaginous protein fraction. (Magnification × 1800.)

REFERENCES

1. **McKenzie, L. S., Horsburgh, B. A., Ghosh, P., and Taylor, T. K. F.,** Osteoarthrosis — the uncertain rationale for anti-inflammatory drug therapy, *Lancet,* 1, 908, 1976.
2. **McKenzie, L. S., Horsburgh, B. A., Ghosh, P., and Taylor, T. K. F.,** Effects of anti-inflammatory drugs on sulphated glycosaminoglycan synthesis in aged human articular cartilage, *Ann. Rheum. Dis.,* 35, 487, 1976.
3. **Palmoski, M. J. and Brandt, K. D.,** Effects of some nonsteroidal anti-inflammatory drugs on proteoglycan metabolism and organisation in canine articular cartilage, *Arthritis Rheum.,* 23, 1010, 1980.
4. **Newman, N. M. and Ling, R. S. M.,** Acetabular bone destruction related to non-steroidal anti-inflammatory drugs, *Lancet,* 2, 11, 1985.
5. **Trnavsky, K. and Trnavsky, Z.,** The influence of phenylbutazone on collagen metabolism in vivo, *Pharmacology,* 6, 9, 1971.
6. **Solomon, L.,** Drug induced arthropathy and necrosis of the femoral head, *J. Bone Jt. Surg.,* 55-B, 246, 1973.
7. **Kalbhen, D. A., Schauer, M., and Wentsche, B.,** Tierexperimentelle Untersuchungen über den Einfluss intra artikular Applizierter Antiphlogistika/Antirheumatika auf den Gelenkknorpel in Vivo, *Z. Rheumaforsch.,* 370, 380, 1978.
8. **Oegema, T. R. and Behrens, F.,** Proteoglycan aggregate synthesis in normal and chronically hydrocortisone-suppressed rabbit articular cartilage, *Arch. Biochem. Biophys.,* 206, 277, 1981.
9. **Chandler, G. N. and Wright, D.,** Deleterious effect of intraarticular hydrocortisone, *Lancet,* 2, 661, 1958.
10. **Higuchi, M. and Abe, K.,** Ultrastructure of the nucleus pulposus in the intervertebral disc after systemic administration of hydrocortisone in mice, *Spine,* 10, 638, 1985.
11. **Taylor, T. K. F. and Akeson, W. H.,** Intervertebral disc prolapse: a review of morphologic and biochemic knowledge concerning the nature of prolapse, *Clin. Orthop. Relat. Res.,* 76, 54, 1970.
12. **Bobechko, W. P. and Hirsch, C.,** Auto-immune response to nucleus pulposus in the rabbit, *J. Bone Jt. Surg.,* 47-B, 574, 1965.
13. **Pankovich, A. M. and Korngold, L.,** A comparison of the antigenic properties of nucleus pulposus and cartilage protein polysaccharide complexes, *J. Immunol.,* 99, 431, 1967.
14. **Malawista, I. and Schubert, M.,** Chondromucoprotein — a new extraction method and alkaline degradation, *J. Biol. Chem.,* 230, 535, 1958.
15. **Elves, M. W., Bucknill, T., and Sullivan, M. F.,** In vitro inhibition of leukocyte migration in patients with intervertebral disc lesions, *Orthop. Clin. North Am.,* 6, 59, 1975.
16. **Gertzbein, S. D., Tile, M., Gross, A., and Falk, R.,** Autoimmunity in degenerative disc disease of the lumbar spine, *Orthop. Clin. North Am.,* 6, 67, 1975.
17. **Gertzbein, S. D., Tait, J. H., and Devlin, S. R.,** The stimulation of lymphocytes by nucleus pulposus in patients with degenerative disc disease of the lumbar spine, *Clin. Orthop. Relat. Res.,* 123, 149, 1977.
18. **Gertzbein, S. D.,** The antigenicity of the intervertebral disc, *Sem. Arthritis Rheum.,* 11(S1), 111, 1981.
19. **Marshall, L. L., Trethewie, E. R., and Curtain, C. C.,** Chemical radiculitis. A clinical, physiological and immunological study, *Clin. Orthop. Relat. Res.,* 129, 61, 1977.
20. **Murphy, R. W.,** Nerve roots and spinal nerves in degenerative disc disease, *Clin. Orthop. Relat. Res.,* 129, 45, 1977.
21. **Radin, E. L. and Bryan, R. S.,** Phenylbutazone for prolapesed discs, *Lancet,* 2, 736, 1968.
22. **Hickey, R. F. J.,** Chronic low back pain. A comparison of diflunisal with paracetamol, *N.Z. Med. J.,* 95, 312, 1982.
23. **Berry, H., Bloom, B., Hamilton, E. B. D., and Swinson, D. R.,** Naproxen, sodium diflunisal and placebo in the treatment of chronic back pain, *Ann. Rheum. Dis.,* 41, 129, 1982.
24. **Ghosh, P., Taylor, T. K. F., and Meachin, A. D.,** A double blind crossover trial of indomethacin, flurbiprofen and placebo in the management of lumbar spondylosis, *Curr. Ther. Res.,* 30, 318, 1981.
25. **Taylor, T. K. F. and Ghosh, P.,** Anti-inflammatory drugs in management of spondylosis, *Br. Med. J.,* 283, 951, 1981.
26. **Taylor, T. K. F., Andrews, J. L., Frost, L. C., Ghosh, P., and Berndt, M. C.,** Glycosaminoglycans, in *Scoliosis Proc. 7th Symp.,* Warner, J. O. and Mehta, M. N., Eds., Praeger, New York, 1985, 23.
27. **Bowness, J. M. and Parkinson, D.,** Increased glycosaminoglycan excretion after chymopapain injection of intervertebral discs, *Clin. Biochem.,* 16, 200, 1983.
28. **Thonar, E. J. M. A., Lenz, M. E., Klintworth, G. K., Caterson, B., Pachman, L. M., Glickman, P., Katz, R., Huff, J., and Kuettner, K. E.,** Quantification of keratan sulfate in blood as a marker of cartilage catabolism, *Arthritis Rheum.,* 28, 1367, 1985.
29. **Heinegard, D., Inerot, S., Wieslander, J., and Lindblad, G.,** A method for the quantification of cartilage proteoglycan structures liberated to the synovial fluid during developing degenerative joint disease, *Scand. J. Clin. Lab. Invest.,* 45, 421, 1985.

30. **Gysen, P., Malaise, M., Gaspar, S., and Franchimont, P.,** Collagenase and protein in synovial fluid in inflammatory and degenerative arthropathies, *Clin. Rheum.,* 4, 39, 1985.

31. **Saxne, T., Heinegard, D., Wollheim, F. A., and Pettersson, H.,** Difference in cartilage proteoglycan level in synovial fluid in early rheumatoid arthritis and reactive arthritis, *Lancet,* July 20, 127, 1985.

32. **Sturrock, R. D. and Hart, F. D.,** Double blind cross-over comparison of indomethacin, flurbiprofen, and placebo in ankylosing spondylitis, *Ann. Rheum. Dis.,* 33, 19, 1974.

33. **Ciocci, A.,** Indomethacin in the treatment of the lumbar disc syndrome, *Inflamm. Arthro.,* 401, 1976.

34. **Coari, G. and Taccari, E.,** Treatment in rheumatology with a new injectable salt of indomethacin, *Minerva Med.,* 65, 917, 1974.

35. **Wasilewski, R. and Tomankiewicz, Z.,** Clinical evaluation of indocid in treatment of acute painful syndromes of radicular origin, *Pol. Tyg. Lek.,* 26, 648, 1971.

36. **Goldie, I.,** A clinical trial with indomethacin (Indomee) in low back pain, *Acta Orthop. Scand.,* 39, 117, 1968.

37. **Nachemson, A.,** Oxyphenbutazone in surgery for herniated discs. A double blind trial, *Acta. Orthop. Scand.,* 37, 267, 1966.

38. **Binzus, G. and Josenhans, G.,** Results of an open therapeutic trial with naproxen in patients with degenerative joint diseases, *Scand. J. Rheumatol.,* 2, 80, 1973.

39. **Ferris, J. E. and Pigott, P. V.,** Evaluation of mefenamic acid and flufenamic acid in clinical pain, *Ann. Phys. Med.,* 84, 1966.

40. **Sorensen, K.,** A long-term investigation of a new antirheumatic drug, diclofenac sodium, *Scand. J. Rheumatol.,* 22, 81, 1978.

41. **Rask, M. R.,** Colchicine use in the damaged disk syndrome. Report of 50 patients, *Clin. Orthop. Relat. Res.,* 143, 183, 1979.

42. **Rask, M. R.,** Colchicine use in disk disorders: report of 300 patients, *J. Neurol. Orthop. Surg.,* 1, 56, 1979.

43. **Rask, M. R.,** Colchicine use in 500 patients with disc disease, *J. Neurol. Orthop. Surg.,* 1, 1, 1980.

44. **Havsy, S. L.,** 110 patients with disc disease, *J. Neurol. Orthop. Med. Surg.,* 5, 221, 1984.

45. **Meek, J. B., Giudice, V. W., and Enrick, N. C.,** Colchicine highly effective in disk disorders: results of a double blind study, *J. Neurol. Orthop. Med. Sur.,* 5, 215, 1984.

46. **Meek, J. B., Giudice, V. W., McFadden, J. W., Key, J. D., and Enrick, N. L.,** Colchicine highly effective in disc disorders, final results of a double blind study, *J. Neurol. Orthop. Med. Surg.,* 6, 211, 1985.

47. **Wallace, S. L.,** Colchicine, in *Textbook of Rheumatology,* Vol. 1, W. B. Saunders, Philadelphia, 1981, chap. 57.

48. **Francis, A. E.,** Theoretical considerations for the use of colchicine (Articulorum) in disc disease, *J. Neurol. Orthop. Med. Surg.,* 7, 235, 1986.

49. **Greenwald, R. A. and Moak, S. A.,** Degradation of hyaluronic-acid by polymorphonuclear leukocytes, *Inflammation,* 10, 15, 1986.

50. **Halliwell, B. and Gutheridge, J. M. C.,** Oxygen toxicity, oxygen radicals, transition metals and disease, *Biochem. J.,* 219, 1, 1984.

51. **Greenwald, R. A. and Moy, W. W.,** Inhibition of collagen gelation by action of the superoxide radical, *Arthritis Rheum.,* 22, 251, 1979.

52. **Greenwald, R. A., Moy, W. W., and Lazarus, D.,** Degradation of cartilage proteoglycans and collagen by superoxide radicals, *Arthritis Rheum.,* 19, 799, 1976.

53. **McCord, J. M. and Wong, K.,** Phagocyte-produced free radicals: roles in cytotoxicity and inflammation, in *Oxygen Free Radicals and Tissue Damage,* Ciba Foundation Symp. 65, Elsevier Excerpta Medica North-Holland, Amsterdam, 1979, 343.

54. **Delmaestro, R. F. and Alexander, I.,** Oxygen derived free radicals: their role in inflammation, in *The Inflammatory Process: An Introduction to the Study of Cellular and Humoral Mechanisms,* Verge, P. and Lindbom, A., Eds., Almqvist & Wiksell International, Stockholm, 1981, 113.

55. **McCord, J. M., Wong, K., Stokes, S. H., Petone, W. F., and English, D.,** Superoxide and inflammation: a mechanism for the anti-inflammatory activity of superoxide desmutase, *Acta Physiol. Scand.,* 492, 25, 1980.

56. **Breshears, D. E., Brown, C. D., Riffel, D. M., Cobble, R. J., and Chessman, S. F.,** Evaluation of orgotein in treatment of locomotor dysfunction in dogs, *Mod. Vet. Pract.,* February, 85, 1974.

57. **Put, T. R.,** The favourable effect of adding a catalase to the treatment of syndromes due to intervertebral disc degenerations, *Arzneim. Forsch.,* 25, 951, 1975.

58. **Polley, H. F. and Slocumb, C. H.,** Behind the scenes with cortisone and ACTH, *Mayo Clin. Proc.,* 51, 471, 1976.

59. **Skidmore, I. F.,** Anti-inflammatory steroids — the pharmacological and biochemical basis of clinical activity, *Mol. Aspects Med.,* 4, 303, 1981.

60. **Fauci, A. S., Dale, D. C., and Balow, J. E.,** Glucocorticosteroid therapy: mechanisms of action and clinical considerations, *Ann. Intern. Med.,* 84, 304, 1976.
61. **Claman, H. N.,** Corticosteroids and lymphoid cells, *N. Engl. J. Med.,* 287, 388, 1972.
62. **Parrillo, J. E. and Fauci, A. S.,** Mechanisms of glucocorticoid action on immune processes, *Annu. Rev. Pharmacol. Toxicol.,* 19, 179, 1979.
63. **Cupps, T. R. and Fauci, A. S.,** Corticosteroid-mediate immunoregulation in man, *Immunol. Rev.,* 65, 133, 1982.
64. **Hofferberth, B., Gottschaldt, M., Grass, H., and Bluttner, K.,** The usefulness of dexamethasone phosphate in the conservative treatment of lumbar pain, a double-blind study, *Arch. Psychiatr. Nervenkr.,* 231, 359, 1982.
65. **Hedeboe, J., Buhl, M., and Ransing, P.,** Effects of using dexamethasone and placebo in the treatment of prolapsed lumbar disc, *Acta Neurol. Scand.,* 65, 6, 1982.
66. **Green, L. N.,** Dexamethasone in the management of symptoms due to herniated lumbar disc, *J. Neurol. Neurosurg. Psychiatr.,* 12, 1211, 1975.
67. **Porsman, O. and Friis, H.,** Lumbar disc prolapse treated with intramuscular injections of dexamethasone (Decadron). Prospective controlled, double-blind study of 52 patients, *Ugeskr. Laeg.,* 142, 2553, 1980.
68. **Porsman, O. and Friis, H.,** Prolapsed lumbar disc treated with intramuscularly administered dexamethasonephosphate. A prospectively planned, double-blind, controlled clinical trial in 52 patients, *Scand. J. Rheumatol.,* 8, 142, 1979.
69. **Sehgal, A. D. and Gardner, W. J.,** Corticosteroids administered intradurally for relief of sciatica, *Cleveland Clin. Q.,* 27, 198, 1960.
70. **Burn, J. M. B. and Langdon, L.,** Lumbar epidural injection for the treatment of chronic sciatica, *Rheumatol. Phys. Med.,* 10, 368, 1970.
71. **Goebert, H. W., Jallo, S. J., Gardner, W. J., Wasmuth, C. E., and Bitte, E. M.,** Sciatica: treatment with epidural injections of procaine and hydrocortisone, *Cleveland Clin. Q.,* 27, 191, 1960.
72. **Mount, H. T.,** Hydrocortisone in the treatment of intervertebral disc protrusion, *Can. Med. Assoc.J.,* 105, 1279, 1971.
73. **Brown, F. W.,** Management of diskogenic pain using epidural and intrathecal steroids, *Clin. Orthop.,* Vol. 129, 72, 1977.
74. **Snoek, W., Weber, H., and Jorgensen, B.,** Double-blind evaluation of extradural methyl prednisolone for herniated lumbar discs, *Acta Orthop. Scand.,* 48, 635, 1977.
75. **Jackson, D. W., Rettig, A., and Wiltse, L. L.,** Epidural cortilone injections in the young athletic adult, *Am. J. Sports Med.,* 8, 239, 1980.
76. **Ryan, M. D. and Taylor, T. K.,** Management of lumbar nerve-root pain by intrathecal and epidural injections of depot methylpredlisolone acetate, *Med. J. Aust.,* 2, 532, 1981.
77. **Harley, C.,** Extradural corticosteroid infiltration. A follow-up study of 50 cases, *Ann. Phys. Med.,* 9, 22, 1967.
78. **Bernat, J. L.,** Intraspinal steroid therapy, *Neurology (New York),* 31, 168, 1981.
79. **Corrigan, A. B., Carr, G., and Tugwell, S.,** Intraspinal corticosteroid injections, *Med. J.,* 1, 224, 1982.
80. **Wood, K. M.,** New approaches to treatment of back pain, *West. J. Med.,* 130, 394, 1979.
81. **Gardner, W. J., Goebert, M. W., and Sehgal, A. D.,** Intraspinal corticosteroid in the treatment of sciatica, *Trans. Am. Neurol. Assoc.,* 86, 214, 1961.
82. **Winnie, A. P., Hartman, J. T., and Meyers, H. L. J.,** Pain clinic. II. Intradural and extradural corticosteroids for sciatica, *Anesth. Analg.,* 51, 990, 1972.
83. **Dilke, T. F. W., Burry, H. C., and Graham, R.,** Extradural corticosteroid injection in management of lumbar nerve root compression, *Br. Med. J.,* 2, 635, 1973.
84. **Fishman, R. A. and Christy, N. P.,** Fate of adrenal cortical steroids following intrathecal injection, *Neurology (Minneapolis),* 15, 1, 1965.
85. **Plumb, V. J. and Dismukes, W. E.,** Chemical meningitis related to intrathecal corticosteroid therapy, *South. Med.,* 70, 1241, 1977.
86. **Feffer, H. L.,** Treatment of low back and sciatic pain by the injection of hydrocortisone into degenerated intervertebral discs, *J. Bone Jt. Surg.,* 38-A, 585, 1956.
87. **Feffer, H. L.,** Therapeutic intradiscal hydrocortisone. A long-term study, *Clin. Orthop.,* 67, 100, 1969.
88. **Feffer, H. L.,** Regional use of steroids in the management of lumbar intervertebral disc disease, *J. Bone Jt. Surg.,* 6, 249, 1975.
89. **Graham, C. E.,** Chemonucleolysis: a double blind study comparing chemonucleolysis with intradiscal hydrocortisone in the treatment of backache and sciatica, *Clin. Orthop. Relat. Res.,* 117, 184, 1976.
90. **Wilkinson, H. A. and Schuman, N.,** Intradiscal corticosteroids in the treatment of lumbar and cervical disc problems, *Spine,* 5, 385, 1980.
91. **Davidson, E. A. and Small, W.,** Metabolism in vivo of connective tissue mucopolysaccharides. I. Chondroitin sulphate C and keratan sulphate of nucleus pulposus, *Biochem. Biolphys. Acta,* 69, 445, 1963.

92. **Silberberg, M., Silberberg, R., and Hasler, M.,** Fine structure of articular cartilage on mice receiving cortisone acetate, *Arch. Pathol.,* 82, 569, 1966.

93. **Barrett, A. J., Sledge, C. B., and Dingle, J. T.,** Effects of cortisol on the synthesis of chondroitin sulphate by embryonic cartilage, *Nature (London),* 211, 83, 1966.

94. **Schryver, H. F.,** The effects of hydrocortisone on chondroitin sulphate production and loss by embryonic chick tibiotarsi in organ culture, *Exp. Cell Res.,* 40, 610, 1965.

95. **Saarni, H. and Hopsu-Havu, V.,** Inhibition of acid mucopolysaccharide synthesis by hydrocortisone, hydrocortisone 17-butyrate and betamethasone 17-valerate, *Br. J. Dermatol.,* 97, 505, 1977.

96. **Paatsama, S., Rissanen, P., and Rokkanen, P.,** Effects of estradiol, testosterone, cortisone acetate, somatotropin, thyrotropin, and parathyroid on the lumbar intervertebral disc in growing dogs, *J. Small Anim. Pract.,* 10, 351, 1969.

97. **Haimovici, E. H.,** Experimental disc lesion in rabbits. The effect of repeated administration, *Acta Orthop. Scand.,* 41, 505, 1970.

98. **Saarni, H. and Hopsu-Havu, V. K.,** Effect of hydrocortisone butyrate on collagen synthesis, *Br. J. Dermatol.,* 95, 566, 1976.

99. **Ebert, P. S. and Prockop, D. J.,** Influence of cortisol on the synthesis of sulphated mucopolysaccharides and collagen in chick embryos, *Biochem. Biophys. Acta,* 136, 45, 1967.

100. **Ott, V. R., Schwenkenbecher, H., and Iser, H.,** Die Spondylose bei Diabetes mellitus, *Z. Rheumaforsch.,* 22, 278, 1963.

101. **Hajkova, Z., Streda, A., and Skrha, F.,** Hyperostotic spondylosis and diabetes mellitus, *Ann. Rheum. Dis.,* 24, 536, 1965.

102. **Forestier, J. and Lagier, R.,** The concept of vertebral ankylosing hyperostosis, *Rev. Rheum.,* 36, 655, 1969.

103. **Forgacs, S.,** Hyperostotische Knochenveranderungen bei Diabetikern, *Radiologe,* 13, 167, 1973.

104. **Silberberg, R. and Gerritsen, G.,** Aging changes in intervertebral discs and spondylosis in Chinese hamsters, *Diabetes,* 25, 477, 1976.

105. **Silberberg, R.,** Vertebral aging in hypopituitary dwarf mice, *Gerontologia,* 19, 281, 1973.

106. **Luft, R. and Guillemin, R.,** Growth hormones and diabetes in man. Old concepts — new implications, *Diabetes,* 23, 783, 1974.

107. **Silberberg, R.,** Response of vertebral cartilage and bone to hormonal imbalances produced by anterior hypothyroidism, *Pathol. Microbiol.,* 41, 11, 1974.

108. **Aufdermaur, M., Fehr, K., Lesker, D., and Silberberg, R.,** Quantitative histochemical changes in intervertebral discs in diabetes, *Exp. Cell Biol.,* 48, 89, 1980.

109. **Hirsch, C.,** Studies on the pathology of low back pain, *J. Bone Jt. Surg.,* 41-B, 237, 1959.

110. **Smith, L.,** Enzyme dissolution of the nucleus pulposus in humans, *J. Am. Med. Assoc.,* 187, 177, 1964.

111. **Thomas, L.,** Reversible collapse of rabbit ears after intravenous papain and prevention of recovery by cortisone, *J. Exp. Med.,* 104, 245, 1956.

112. **Smith, L., Garvin, P. J., Gesler, R. M., and Jennings, R. B.,** Enzyme dissolution of the nucleus pulposus, *Nature (London),* 198, 4887, 1963.

113. **Garvin, P. J., Jennings, R. B., Smith, L., and Gesler, R. M.,** Chymopapain: a pharmacologic and toxicologic evaluation in experimental animals, *Clin. Orthop.,* 41, 204, 1965.

114. **Gesler, R. M.,** Pharmacological properties of chymopapain, *Clin. Orthop. Relat. Res.,* 67, 47, 1969.

115. **Branemark, P. I., Ekholm, R., and Lundskog, J.,** Tissue response to chymopapain in different concentrations. Animal investigations on microvascular effects, *Clin. Orthop. Relat. Res.,* 67, 52, 1969.

116. **Arnon, R.,** Papain, in Proteolytic enzymes, Perlmann, G. E. and Lorand, L., Eds., *Methods Enzymol.,* 19, 243, 1970.

117. **Stern, I. J., Cosmas, F., and Smith, L.,** Urinary polyuronide excretion in man after enzymic dissolution of the chondromucoprotein of the intervertebral disc or surgical stress, *Clin. Chem.,* 21, 181, 1968.

118. **Stern, I. J.,** Biochemistry of chymopapain, *Clin. Orthop. Relat. Res.,* 67, 42, 1969.

119. **Garvin, P. J., Jennings, R. B., and Stern, I. J.,** Enzymic digestion of the nucleus pulposus: a review of experimental studies with chymopapain, *Orthop. Clin. North Am.,* 8, 27, 1977.

120. **Artigas, J., Brock, M., and Mayer, H.-M.,** Complications following chemonucleolysis with collagenase, *J. Neurosurg.,* 61, 679, 1984.

121. **Garvin, P. J. and Jennings, R. B.,** Long-term effects of chymopapain on intervertebral disks of dogs, *Clin. Orthop. Relat. Res.,* 92, 281, 1973.

122. **Kapsalis, A. A., Stern, I. J., and Bornstein, I.,** The fate of chymopapain injected for therapy of intervertebral disc disease, *J. Lab. Clin. Med.,* 83, 532, 1974.

123. **Bradford, D. S., Cooper, K. M., and Oegema, T. R.,** Chymopapain, chemonucleolysis, and nucleus pulposus regeneration, *J. Bone Jt. Surg.,* 65-A, 1220, 1983.

124. **Bradford, D. S., Oegema, T. R., Cooper, K. M., Wakano, K., and Chao, E. Y.,** Chymopapain, chemonucleolysis and nucleus pulposus regeneration: a biochemical and biomechanical study, *Spine,* 9, 135, 1984.

125. **Braund, K. G., Ghosh, P., Taylor, T. K. F., and Larsen, L. H.,** Morphological studies of the canine intervertebral disc. The assignment of the beagle to the achondroplastic classification, *Res. Vet. Sci.,* 19, 167, 1975.

126. **Hansen, H.-J.,** A pathological anatomical study on disc degeneration in dog, *Acta Orthop. Scand. Suppl.,* 11, 9, 1952.

127. **Ghosh, P., Taylor, T. K. F., Braund, K. G., and Larsen, L.H.,** The collagenous and non-collaginous proteins of the canine intervertebral disc and their variation with age, spinal level and breed, *Gerontolgia,* 22, 124, 1976.

128. **Ghosh, P., Taylor, T. K. F., Braund, K. G., and Larsen, L.H.,** A comparative chemical and histo-chemical study of the chondrodystrophoid canine intervertebral disc, *Vet. Pathol.,* 13, 414, 1976.

129. **Ghosh, P., Taylor, T. K. F., and Braund, K. G.,** Variation of the glycosaminoglycans of the canine intervertebral disc with aging. I. Chondrodystrophoid breed, *Gerontology,* 23, 87, 1977.

130. **Ghosh, P., Taylor, T. K. F., and Braund, K. G.,** Variation of the glycosaminoglycans of the canine intervertebral disc with aging. II. Non-chondrodystrophoid breed, *Gerontology,* 23, 99, 1977.

131. **Kahanovits, N., Arnoczky, S. P., and Kummer, F.,** The comparative biomechanical, histologic, and radiographic analysis of canine lumbar discs treated by surgical excision or chemonucleolysis, *Spine,* 10, 178, 1985.

132. **Trout, J. J., Buckwalter, J. A., and Moore, K. C.,** Ultrastructure of the human intervertebral disc. II. Cells of the nucleus pulposus, *Anat. Rec.,* 204, 307, 1982.

133. **Widdowson, W. L.,** Effects of chymopapain in the intervertebral disc of the dog, *J. Am. Vet. Med. Assoc.,* 150, 608, 1967.

134. **Shealy, C. N.,** Tissue reactions of chymopapain in cats, *J. Neurosurg.,* 26, 327, 1967.

135. **Ford, L. T.,** Experimental studies of chymopapain in cats, *Clin. Orthop.,* 67, 68, 1969.

136. **Cockayne, D., Willatt, J. E., Buttle, D. J., and Day, S.,** Relative activity and stability of commercially available chymopapain formulations from chemonucleolysis, in *Current Concepts in Chemonucleolysis,* Sutton, J. C., Ed., Royal Society of Medicine, International Congress Symposium Series, 72, 1985, 9.

137. **Zook, B. C. and Kobrine, A. I.,** Effects of collagenase and chymopapain on spinal nerves and intervertebral disc of cynomolgus monkeys, *J. Neurosurg.,* 64, 474, 1986.

138. **Rhodes, R. K.,** Blood vessels, in *Collagen in Health and Disease,* Weiss, J. B. and Jayson, M. I. V., Eds., Churchill Livingstone, Edinburgh, 1982, 376.

139. **Werb, Z.,** Degradation of collagen, in *Collagen in Health and Disease,* Weiss, J. B. and Jayson, M. I. V., Eds., Churchill Livingstone, Edinburgh, 1982, 121.

140. **Wiltse, L. L., Widell, E. H., Jr., and Yuan, H. A.,** Chymopapain chemonucleolysis in lumbar disc disease, *J. Am. Med. Assoc.,* 231, 474, 1975.

141. **Wiltse, L. L.,** Chemonucleolysis in the treatment of lumbar disc disease, *Orthop. Clin. North Am.,* 14, 605, 1983.

142. **McCulloch, J. A.,** Chemonucleolysis. Experience with 2000 cases, *Clin. Orthop. Relat. Res.,* 146, 128, 1980.

143. **Sussman, B. J.,** Inadequacies and hazards of chymopapain injections as treatment for intervertebral disc disease, *J. Neurosurg.,* 42, 389, 1975.

144. **Di Maio, V. J.,** Two anaphylactic deaths after chemonucleolysis, *J. Forensic Sci.,* 21, 187, 1976.

145. **Moneret-Vautrin, D. A. and Laxenaire, M. C.,** Anaphylaxis to purified chymopapain, in *Current Concepts in Chemonucleolysis,* Sutton, J. C., Ed., Royal Society of Medicine, International Congress Symposium Series, 72, 1985, 77.

146. **Mayer, H. M. and Brock, M.,** Chymopapain allergy. Diagnostic value of a skin test before and after chemonucleolysis, *Neurochirurgis (Stuttgart),* 28, 51, 1985.

147., **Tsay, Y. G., Jones, R., Calenoff, E., Sun, J., Arndt, L., Crispin, B., and Rock, H.,** A preoperative chymopapain sensitivity test for chemonucleolysis candidates, *Spine,* 9, 764, 1984.

148. **Dyke, P.,** Paraplegia following chemonucleolysis: a case report and discussion of neurotoxicity, *Spine,* 10, 359, 1985.

149. **Debb, Z. L., Schimel, S., Daffner, R. H., Lupetin, A. R., Hryshko, F. G., and Blakley, J. B.,** Intervertebral disk-space infection after chympapain injection, *Am. J. Neuroradiol.,* 6, 55, 1985.

150. **Brian, J. E., Jr., Westerman, G. R., and Chadduck, W. M.,** Septic complications of chemonucleolysis, *Neurosurgery,* 15, 730, 1984.

151. **Saunders, E. C.,** Treatment of the intervertebral disc syndrome by direct injection of an enzyme, *J. Am. Vet. Med. Assoc.,* 145, 896, 1964.

152. **Smith, L. and Brown, J. E.,** Treatment of lumbar intervertebral disc lesions by direct injection of chymopapain, *J. Bone Jt. Surg.,* 49, 502, 1967.

153. **Martins, A. N., Ramirez, A., Johnston, J. and Schwetschenau, P. R.,** Double-blind evaluation of chemonucleolysis for herniated lumbar discs. Late results, *J. Neurosurg.,* 49, 816, 1978.

154. **Brown, J. E.,** Clinical studies on chemonucleolysis, *Clin. Orthop. Relat. Res.,* 67, 94, 1969.

155. **Brown, M. D.,** Chemonucleolysis with discase: technique, results, case reports, *Spine*, 1, 115, 1976.
156. **Day, P. L.,** Lateral approach for lumbar discogram and chemonucleolysis, *Clin. Orthop. Relat. Res.*, 67, 90, 1969.
157. **Day, P. L.,** Early, interim and long term observations on chemonucleolysis in 876 patients with special comments on the lateral approach, *Clin. Orthop. Relat. Res.*, 99, 64, 1974.
158. **Ford, L. T.,** Clinical use of chymopapain in lumbar and dorsal disc lesions, *Clin. Orthop. Relat. Res.*, 67, 81, 1969.
159. **Graham, C. E.,** Backache and sciatica: a report of 90 patients treated by intradiscal injection of chymopapain (Discase), *Med. J. Aust.*, 1, 5, 1974.
160. **Herrock, R. B., Daughety, J. S., and Hoover, B. B.,** Clinical and electromyographic evaluation after chemonucleolysis for lumbar disc disease, *South. Med. J.*, 682, 1552, 1975.
161. **Javid, M. J.,** Treatment of herniated lumbar disc syndrome with chymopapain, *J. Am. Med. Assoc.*, 243, 2043, 1980.
162. **MacNab, I.,** Chemonucleolysis, *Clin. Neurosurg.*, 20, 183, 1973.
163. **Maroon, J. C., Hoist, R. A., and Osgood, C. P.,** Chymopapain in the treatment of ruptured lumbar discs: preliminary experiments in 48 patients, *J. Neurol. Neurosurg. Psychiatr.*, 39, 508, 1976.
164. **McCulloch, J. A.,** Chemonucleolysis, *J. Bone Jt. Surg.*, 59-B, 45, 1977.
165. **Schoedinger, G. R. and Ford, L. T.,** The use of chymopapain in ruptured lumbar discs, *South. Med. J.*, 64, 333, 1071.
166. **MacNab, I., McCulloch, J. A., Weiner, D. S., Hugo, E. P., Galway, R. D., and Dall, D.,** Chemonucleolysis, *Can. J. Surg.*, 14, 280, 1971.
167. **McNeill, T., Huncke, B., and Pesch, R. N.,** Chemonucleolysis. Evaluation of effectiveness by electromyography, *Arch. Phys. Med. Rehabil.*, 58, 303, 1977.
168. **Nordby, E. J. and Brown, M. D.,** Present status of chymopapain and chemonucleolysis, *Clin. Orthop.*, 129, 79, 1977.
169. **Onofrio, B. M.,** Injection of chymopapain into intervertebral discs: preliminary report on 72 patients with symptoms of disc disease, *J. Neurosurg.*, 42, 384, 1975.
170. **Parkinson, D. and Shield, C.,** Treatment of protruded lumbar intervetebral discs with chymopapain (Discase), *J. Neurosurg.*, 39, 203, 1973.
171. **Parkinson, D.,** Late results of treatment of intervertebral disc disease with chymopapain, *J. Neurosurg.*, 59, 990, 1983.
172. **Smith, L. and Brown, J. E.,** Treatment of lumbar intervertebral disc lesions by direct injection of chymopapain, *J. Bone Jt. Surg.*, 49-B, 502, 1967.
173. **Sullivan, M.,** Chemonucleolysis, *Proc. R. Soc. Med.*, 68, 479, 1975.
174. **Watts, C., Knighton, R., and Roulhac, G.,** Chymopapain treatment of intervertebral disc disease, *J. Neurosurg.*, 42, 374, 1975.
175. **Weiner, D. S. and MacNab, I.,** The use of chymopapain in degenerative disc disease: a preliminary report, *Can. Med. Assoc. J.*, 102, 1252, 1970.
176. **Simmons, J. W., Stavinoha, W. B., and Knodel, L. C.,** Update and review of chemonucleolysis, *Clin. Orthop. Relat. Res.*, 183, 51, 1984.
177. **Watts, C.,** Chemonucleolysis: an appeal for objectivity, *J. Neurosurg.*, 42, 488, 1975.
178. **Ford, L. T.,** Chymopapain — past, present future?, *Clin. Orthop.*, 122, 367, 1977.
179. **Sampson, P.,** Chymopapain: a case study in federal drug regulation, *J. Am. Med. Assoc.*, 240, 195, 1978.
180. **Gunby, P.,** Chymopapain: tropical tree to surgical suite, *J. Am. Med. Assoc.*, 249, 1115, 1983.
181. **Fager, C. A.,** The age-old back problem: new fad, same fallacies, *Spine*, 9, 326, 1984.
182. **Brown, M. D. and Daroff, R. B.,** The double blind study comparing discase to placebo. An editorial comment, *Spine*, 2, 233, 1977.
183. **Schwetschenau, P. R., Ramirez, A., Johnston, J., Wiggs, C., and Martins, A. N.,** Double-blind evaluation of intradiscal chymopapain for herniated lumbar discs. Early results, *J. Neurosurg.*, 45, 622, 1976.
184. **Javid, M. J., Nordby, E. J., Ford, L. T., Hejna, W. J., Whistler, W. W., Burton, C., Millett, K., Wiltse, L. L., Widell, E. H., Boyd, R. J., Newton, S. E., and Thisted, R.,** Safety and efficacy of chymopapain (chymodiactin) in herniated nucleus pulposus with sciatica, *J. Am. Med. Assoc.*, 249, 2489, 1983.
185. **Nordby, E. J. and Lucas, G. L.,** A comparative analysis of lumbar disk disease treated by laminectomy or chemonucleolysis, *Clin. Orthop.*, 90, 119, 1973.
186. **Watts, C., Hutchison, G., Stern, J., and Clark, K.,** Comparison of intervertebral disc disease treatment by chymopapain injection and open surgery, *J. Neurosurg.*, 42, 397, 1975.
187. **Dabezies, E. J. and Brunet, M.,** Chemonucleolysis versus laminectomy, *Orthopaedics*, 1, 26, 1978.
188. **Sorbie, C. S.,** Chemonucleolysis in the treatment of lumbar disc protrusion, *Can. Med. Assoc. J.*, 124, 840, 1981.

189. **Fraser, R. D.,** Chymopapain for the treatment of intervertebral disc herniation: a preliminary report of a double-blind study, *Spine*, 7, 608, 1982.

190. **Fraser, R. D.,** Chymopapain for the treatment of intervertebral disc herniation: the final report of a double-blind study, *Spine*, 9, 815, 1984.

191. **Mcdermott, D. J., Agre, K., Brim, M., Demma, F. J., Nelson, J., Wilson, R. R., and Thisted, R. A.,** Chymodiactin in patients with herniated lumbar intervertebral disc(s): an open-label, multicenter study, *Spine*, 10, 242, 1985.

192. **Ejeslar, A., Nachemson, A., Herberts, P., Lysell, E., Andersson, G., Irstam, L., and Peterson, L.-E.,** Surgery versus chemonucleolysis for herniated lumbar discs: a prospective study with random assignment, *Clin. Orthop. Relat. Res.*, 174, 236, 1983.

193. **Crawshaw, C., Frazer, A. M., Merriam, W. F., Mulholland, R. C., and Webb, J. K.,** A comparison of surgery and chemonucleolysis in the treatment of sciatica. A prospective randomized trial, *Spine*, 9, 195, 1984.

194. **Taylor, T. K. F. and Ghosh, P.,** Tropical fruit in the treatment of lumbar disc prolapse, *Med. J.*, 142, 462, 1985.

195. **Dunlop, R. B., Adams, M. A., and Hutton, W. C.,** Disc space narrowing and the lumbar facet joints, *J. Bone Jt. Surg.*, 66, 706, 1984.

196. **Watts, C.,** Use of chymopapain in children, *J. Neurosurg.*, 59, 1108, 1983.

197. **Lorenz, M. and McCulloch, J.,** Chemonucleolysis for herniated nucleus pulposus in adolescents, *J. Bone Jt. Surg.*, 67-A, 1402, 1985.

198. **Weber, H.,** Lumbar disc herniation: a controlled prospective study with ten years of observation, *Spine*, 8, 131, 1983.

199. **Watts, C.,** Mechanism of action of chymopapain in ruptured lumbar disc disease, *Clin. Neurosurg.*, 30, 642, 1983.

200. **Murphy, F.,** Sources and patterns of pain in disc disease, *Clin. Neurosurg.*, 15, 343, 1968.

201. **McCulloch, J. A. and MacNab, I.,** *Sciatica and Chymopapain,* Waverley Press, Baltimore, Md., 100, 1983.

202. **MacNab, I. and McCulloch, J. A.,** Chemonucleolysis, *Can. J. Surg.*, 14, 180, 1971.

203. **Krempen, J. F., Minnig, D. I., and Smith, B. S.,** Experimental studies on the effect of chymopapain on nerve root compression caused by intervertebral disk material, *Clin. Orthop. Relat. Res.*, 106, 336, 1975.

204. **MacKinnon, S. E., Hudson, A. R., Llamao, F., Dellon, A. L., Kline, D. G., and Hunter, D. A.,** Peripheral nerve injury by chymopapain injections, *J. Neurosurg.*, 61, 1, 1984.

205. **Sussman, B. J.,** Intervertebral discolysis with collagenase, *Lancet*, 2, 815, 1967.

206. **Sussman, B. J.,** Intervertebral discolysis with collagenase, *J. Natl. Med. Assoc.*, 60, 184, 1968.

207. **Sussman, B. J. and Mann, M.,** Experimental intervertebral discolysis with collagenase, *J. Neurosurg.*, 31, 628, 1969.

208. **Bromley, J. W., Hirst, J. W., Osman, M., Steinlauf, P., Gennace, R. E., and Stern, H.,** Collagenase: an experimental study of intervertebral disc dissolution, *Spine*, 5, 126, 1980.

209. **Garvin, P. J.,** Toxicity of collagenase: the relation to enzyme therapy of disk herniation, *Clin. Orthop. Relat. Res.*, 101, 286, 1974.

210. **Stern, W. E. and Coulson, W. F.,** Effects of collagenase upon the intervertebral disc in monkeys, *J. Neurosurg.*, 44, 32, 1976.

211. **Rydevik, B., Brown, M. D., Ehira, T., and Nordborg, C.,** Effects of collagenase on nerve tissue. An experimental study on acute and long-term effects in rabbits, *Spine*, 10, 562, 1985.

212. **Mandl, I.,** Collagenase, *Science*, 169, 1234, 1970.

213. **Bond, M. D. and Van Wart, H. E.,** Purification and separation of individual collagenases of *Clostridium histolyticum* using red dye ligand chromotography, *Biochem.*, 23, 3077, 1984.

214. **Sussman, B. J., Bromley, J. W., and Gomez, J. C.,** Injection of collagenase in the treatment of herniated lumbar disk: initial clinical report, *J. Am. Med. Assoc.*, 245, 730, 1981.

215. **Gomez, J. G., Patino, R., and Lopez, P.,** Lumbar discolysis with collagenase, *Neurol. Colomb.*, 5, 658, 1981.

216. **Bromley, J. W. and Gomez, J. G.,** Lumbar intervertebral discolysis with collagenase, *Spine*, 8, 322, 1983.

217. **Bromley, J. W., Varma, A. O., Santoro, A. J., Cohen, P., Jacobs, R., and Berger, L.,** Double-blind evaluation of collagenase injections for herniated lumbar discs, *Spine*, 9, 486, 1984.

218. **Brock, M., Roggendorf, W., Gorge, H. H., and Curio, G.,** Severe local tissue lesions after chemonucleolysis with collagenase, *Surg. Neurol.*, 22, 124, 1984.

219. **Sussman, B. J.,** Effect of collagenase on monkey intervertebral discs (letter), *J. Neurosurg.*, 44, 767, 1976.

220. **Avakian, A. V.,** The effects of the proteolytic enzymes trypsin and chymopsin on intervertebral disks under experimental conditions, *Eksp. Khir. Anesteziol.*, 17, 23, 1972.

221. **Gol, A., Andrews, R. F., and Manicom, R. E.,** Treatment of disc lesions of the lumbar spine by intradisk injections of enzymes, *South. Med. J.,* 59, 1293, 1966.
222. **Oegema, T. R., Swedenburg, S. M., and Bradford, D. S.,** Biological effects of proteases on dog intervertebral disc, *Trans. Orthop. Soc.,* 2, 423, 1986.
223. **Kramer, J. and Laturnus, H.,** Treatment of lumbar intervertebral disc lesions by intradiscal instillation of pressure reducing substances (transl.), *Z. Orthop.,* 113, 1031, 1975.
224. **Kraemer, J. and Laturnus, H.,** Lumbar instillation with aprotinin, *Spine,* 7, 73, 1982.
225. **Lesoin, F., Jomin, M., Viaud, C., Lozes, G., Pruvo, J. P., and Clarisse, J.,** Cervical intradiskal injection of aprotinin. Technical note and preliminary report, *Surg. Neurol.,* 21, 539, 1984.
226. **Ghosh, P., Andrews, J. L., Osborne, R., and Lesjak,M.,** Variations with aging and degeneration of serine and cysteine proteinase inhibitors of human articular cartilage, *Agents Actions,* S18, 69, 1986.
227. **Nakagawa, T., Ghosh, P., and Nagai, Y.,** Serine proteinase and serine proteinase inhibitors of normal and degenerate knee joint menisci, *Biomed. Res.,* 4, 25, 1983.
228. **Cole, T.-C., Burkhardt, D., Frost, L., and Ghosh, P.,** The proteoglycans of the canine intervertebral disc, *Biochim. Biophys. Acta,* 839, 127, 1985.
229. **Cole, T.-C., Ghosh, P., and Taylor, T. K. F.,** Variation of the proteoglycans of the canine intervertebral with ageing, *Biochim. Biophys. Acta,* 880, 209, 1986.
230. **Melrose, J., Ghosh, P., and Taylor, T. K. F.,** Neutral proteinases of the intervertebral disc, *Biochim. Biophys. Acta.,* 923, 483, 1987.
231. **Cole, T-C., Ghosh, P., and Taylor, T. K. F.,** Reduced degradation of disc proteoglycans in vivo, by systemic administration of Arteparon, *J. Bone Jt. Surg.,* 69B, in press.
232. **Hofmann, H. F.,** Arteparon. A basic agent for the therapy of arthrosis, *Therapiewoche,* 31, 7131, 1981.
233. **Baici, A., Salgam, P., Fehr, K., and Boni, A.,** Inhibition of human elastase from polymorphonuclear leucocytes by a glycosaminoglycan polysulphate (Arteparon), *Biochem. Pharmacol.,* 29, 1723, 1980.
234. **Stephens, R. W., Walton, E. A., and Ghosh, P.,** Radioassay for proteolytic cleavage of isolated proteoglycans. The inhibition of human elastase and cathepsin G by anti-inflammatory drugs, *Arzneim. Forsch.,* 30, 2108, 1980.
235. **Andrew, J. L., Sutherland, J., and Ghosh, P.,** Distribution and binding of glycosaminoglycan polysulphate to intervertebral disc, knee joint articular cartilage and meniscus, *Arzneim. Forsch.,* 35, 144, 1985.
236. **Greiling, H. and Kaneko, M.,** Die hemmung lysosomaler Enzyme durch ein Glykosaminoglykan Polysulfat, *Arnzeim. Forsch.,* 23, 593, 1973.
237. **Caterson, B., Christner, J. E., Baker, J. R., and Couchman, J. R.,** Production and characterisation of monoclonal antibodies directed against connective tissue proteoglycans, *Fed. Proc.,* 44, 386, 1985.
238. **Dapas, F., Hartman, S. F., Martinez, L., Northrup, B. E., Nussdorf, R. T., Silberman, H. M., and Gross, H.,** Baclofen for the treatment of acute low-back syndrome, *Spine,* 10, 345, 1985.
239. **Bain, L. S.,** The use of diazepam in the treatment of musculoskeletal disorders, *Ann. Phys. Med.,* Suppl., 3, 1964.
240. **Hingorani, K.,** Diazepam in backache. A double-blind controlled trial, *Ann. Phys. Med.,* 8, 303, 1966.
241. **Feffer, H. L.,** Double-blind evaluation of diazepam, sodium pentobarbital, and placebo as adjunctive premedicants prior to discography, *Clin. Orthop.,* 100, 242, 1974.
242. **Gaspardy, G., Balint, G., Mitusova, M., and Lorincz, G.,** Treatment of sciatica due to intervertebral disc herniation with chymoral tablets, *Rheumatol. Phys. Med.,* 11, 14, 1971.
243. **Gibson, T., Dilke, T. F., and Grahame, R.,** Chymoral in the treatment of lumbar disc prolapse, *Rheumatol. Rehabil.,* 14, 186, 1975.
244. **Auld, A. W., Perlmutter, M. D., and Dooley, D. M.,** Use of urea in the herniated intervertebral disc syndrome, *J. Florida Med. Ass.,* 56, 181, 1969.
245. **Steinberg, A.,** The employment of dimethyl sulfoxide as an anti-inflammatory agent and steroid-transporter in diversified clinical diseases, *Ann. N.Y. Acad. Sci.,* 141, 532, 1967.
246. **Alfonsi, E., Berzero, G. F., Zandrini, C., and Felicetti, G.,** The role of drug therapy in the treatment of nerve root lesions caused by compression. Clinical and electrophysiological study of 30 patients operated on for the removal of herniated disks, *Minerva Med.,* 75, 1727, 1984.

Chapter 13

POTENTIAL OF MAGNETIC RESONANCE IMAGING FOR THE INVESTIGATION OF DISC PATHOLOGY

David W. L. Hukins, Richard M. Aspden, and D. Stephen Hickey

TABLE OF CONTENTS

I. INTRODUCTION

Magnetic resonance (MR) is increasingly being used as a noninvasive method for clinical imaging of the spine and, in particular, for investigating the pathology of the intervertebral disc.[1,2] The technique yields an image of a cross section of the body; a brief introduction to the kind of structural information it can provide on the disc is included in Chapter 1, Volume 1. The present chapter gives a much more detailed account of the principles of magnetic resonance imaging so that its potential for experimental and clinical investigation of disc degeneration can be discussed further.

MR imaging exploits the phenomenon of nuclear magnetic resonance (NMR) which was discovered in 1946 by Bloch et al.,[3] and independently by Purcell et al.;[4] the application of NMR to imaging was successfully developed from about 1973,[5,6] although its potential for providing spatial information appears to have been recognized for a long time.[7,8] Unfortunately the nomenclature can be confusing; MR imaging, MRI, NMR imaging, and zeugmatography all refer to exactly the same technique. Physicists tend to refer to "nuclear magnetic resonance," rather than simple "magnetic resonance," to distinguish it from "electron paramagnetic resonance" (also called "electron spin resonance"); however, it is only NMR which so far has been applied to clinical imaging, and so reference to "magnetic resonance imaging" is unambiguous.

Only certain nuclei exhibit NMR; the most common is the hydrogen nucleus, which consists of a single proton. (Hence the occasional reference, in the literature, to proton magnetic resonance, or PMR, which refers specifically to NMR of hydrogen nuclei.) Further examples of nuclei which exhibit NMR, together with the natural abundance of the isotope each represents in the naturally occurring element and in the human body, are listed in Table 1. So far MR imaging of the spine has been restricted to hydrogen nuclei, which, in the disc, are mostly present in water molecules. Thus, for the purposes of this chapter, an MR image provides information about the hydrogen nuclei or, more specifically, about the water molecules in the intervertebral disc.

The aim of this chapter is to show how MR imaging can be exploited for the investigation of disc degeneration and aging. Since the technique can do more than just provide pictures of the tissues, it will be necessary to describe some of the principles involved. Section II presents these principles at the most elementary level appropriate to understanding Sections IV and V. Further details are presented in Section III, which also discusses some concepts which may prove important in future applications of the technique to the disc; however, this section may be skipped without loss of continuity. More information on the principles and further justification for many of the statements made in Sections II and III are given elsewhere.[9-13]

II. MR IMAGING: A BRIEF INTRODUCTION

A. Nuclear Magnetic Resonance

A bar magnet, which is free to move, will align itself in a magnetic field; thus a compass needle aligns itself in the earth's field and points toward the magnetic north pole. However, if the magnet is spinning about its axis, its behavior in an external magnetic field is much more complicated. Figure 1 shows that it then precesses about the field direction, i.e., as well as spinning about its axis, one end moves around the field direction in a circular path. This circular path is indicated by a dashed line in the figure. The motion of the spinning magnet in the external field is exactly the same as that of a spinning top (or a gyroscope) in the earth's gravitational field.

Nuclei listed in Table 1 are effectively spinning magnets, as shown in Figure 2a, and so the axes of all these magnetic nuclei will precess about the direction of an applied magnetic

Table 1
EXAMPLES OF NUCLEI WHICH EXHIBIT
NMR WITH THEIR NATURAL ABUNDANCE
AND THE APPROXIMATE NUMBER OF
NUCLEI OF EACH ISOTOPE IN THE BODY
RELATIVE TO HYDROGEN

Isotope	Natural abundance (%)	Relative No. of nuclei
^{1}H	99.98	1
^{13}C	1.11	0.0015
^{23}Na	100	0.0006
^{31}P	100	0.003

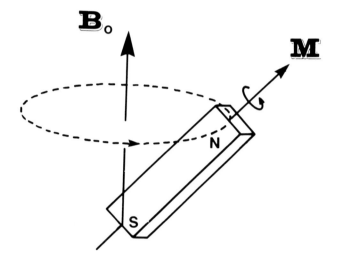

FIGURE 1. A bar magnet which is spinning about its axis will precess about the direction of an applied magnetic field, B_o, as shown.

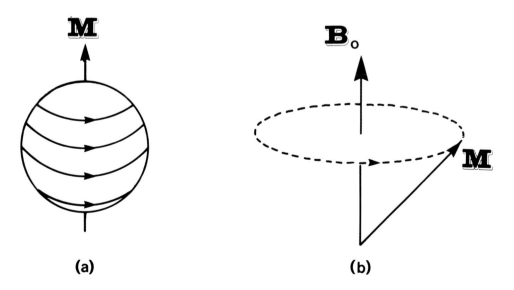

(a)   **(b)**

FIGURE 2. Since (a) the magnetic nucleus is effectively a spinning magnet, it will precess about the direction of an applied magnetic field, B_o, as shown in (b) by analogy with Figure 1.

Table 2
VALUES FOR THE
MAGNETIC RATIO,
γ, OF THE
ISOTOPES LISTED
IN TABLE 1

Isotope	γ(rad/Tsec)
^1H	2.68×10^8
^{13}C	0.67×10^8
^{23}Na	2.13×10^8
^{31}P	1.08×10^8

field as shown in Figure 2b. The natural frequency for this precession, sometimes called the "Larmor frequency," is given by

$$\nu_0 = \gamma B_0/2\pi \tag{1}$$

where B_o is the magnetic flux density (measured in tesla, T) and γ is a constant for a given type of nucleus (see Table 2) called its magnetogyric (or gyromagnetic) constant. This frequency can be imagined as the number of times that one end of the axis of the nucleus passes around the circular path (dashed) of Figure 2b; the frequency is then given in hertz (Hz), but a more convenient measure is the megahertz (MHz), where 1 MHz is identical to 10^6 Hz.

For example, the Larmor frequency for hydrogen nuclei in a 0.26-T magnetic field can be calculated as follows:

$$\nu_0 = 2.68 \times 10^8 \times 0.26/2\pi = 11 \text{ MHz} \tag{2}$$

(using the appropriate value for γ from Table 2 in Equation 1) i.e., the hydrogen nuclei precess about the direction of the applied field 11,000,000 times a second. Sometimes an angular frequency, ω, is specified so that the natural frequency is given by

$$\omega_0 = 2\pi\nu_0 = \gamma B_0 \tag{3}$$

In our example the angular natural frequency is then simply

$$\omega_0 = 2.68 \times 10^8 \times 0.26 = 7.0 \times 10^7 \text{ rad/sec} \tag{4}$$

Each type of magnetic nucleus thus has its own characteristic Larmor frequency in a given strength of magnetic field.

Such a system can absorb electromagnetic radiation whose frequency is equal to its Larmor frequency; this phenomenon is called nuclear magnetic resonance. NMR occurs because the radiation can transfer its energy to the system provided it has the correct (natural) frequency. It can be most simply explained by analogy with a simple mechanical system — pushing a child on a swing. This system has a natural, resonant frequency (usually about 0.5 Hz), and the child can be helped to swing higher (i.e., the system can be supplied with more energy) provided it is pushed at this frequency. Pushing at the wrong frequency will tend to impair the motion of the swing. Similarly the magnetic field associated with the electromagnetic radiation can only provide the precessing nuclear magnets with energy if its frequency corresponds to the natural frequency (i.e., the Larmor frequency) of the system.

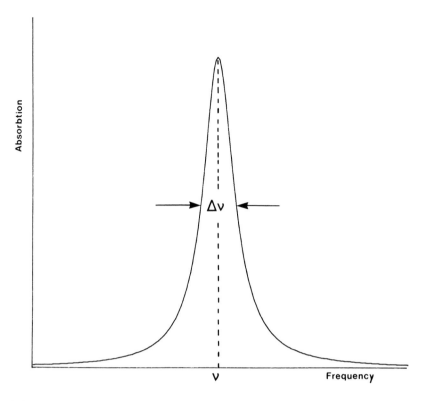

FIGURE 3.   Absorption of radiowaves by a sample containing magnetic nuclei as a function of frequency, ν, where ν_0 is the Larmor frequency and $\Delta\nu$ is the width of the absorption peak at half its maximum height.

Thus, hydrogen nuclei in a magnetic field of 0.26 T can absorb electromagnetic radiation with a frequency of 11 MHz, according to Equation 2; this corresponds to a radio frequency (RF; e.g., BBC Radio 1 transmits at 1.1 MHz). NMR phenomena are thus characterized by the absorption of radio waves by materials in a magnetic field. Furthermore, by choosing the correct frequency for the radiation, the type of nucleus to be investigated can be selected. Experiments on the intervertebral disc have so far been confined to hydrogen nuclei because they are present in far greater quantity than any of the other nuclei which exhibit the NMR phenomenon (see Table 1 for a list of some common nuclei which exhibit NMR).

B. Relaxation Times

RF radiation whose frequency, ν, is very close to the Larmor frequency, ν_0, may also be absorbed — but not so strongly. To return to the analogy of the child on the swing, pushing at roughly the natural frequency will help — but not as much as pushing at exactly the correct frequency. Figure 3 shows how the absorption depends on ν and defines the width, $\Delta\nu$, of the absorption peak. For an absorbing hydrogen nucleus in the intervertebral disc $\Delta\nu$ may be as narrow as 10 Hz, which means that the range of frequencies which can be absorbed is typically very small. Strictly $\Delta\nu$ is the width of the peak, centered at ν_0, at half its maximum height.

According to the theory of NMR, $\Delta\nu$ depends on how rapidly a precessing nucleus, like that in Figure 2b, can pass its energy on to other similar nuclei around it. The time which it takes for energy to be passed on by this mechanism is called the spin-spin relaxation time, T_2, and is related to $\Delta\nu$ by

$$\Delta\nu = 1/(\pi T_2) \tag{5}$$

In practice, other processes may further broaden the absorption peak so that the observed width, Δv^*, is greater than Δv. Sometimes an empirical relaxation time, T_2^*, is defined by

$$T_2^* = 1/(\pi \Delta v^*) \tag{6}$$

Since Δv^* is greater than Δv, T_2^* must be less than T_2.

A further relaxation time, called the spin-lattice relaxation time, T_1, does not affect the width of the absorption peak. T_1 is a measure of the time that a precessing nucleus takes to dissipate its energy to surrounding molecules. Thus the values of T_1 and T_2 depend on the surroundings of the molecules which contain the precessing nuclei. It is worth noting that, in biological systems, T_1 is invariably greater than T_2^* and, hence, than T_2;[12] for hydrogen nuclei in the nucleus pulposus of a healthy young disc $T_1 \simeq 900$ msec while $T_2 \simeq 200$ msec.[14]

C. Proton Density

Since the area under the peak in Figure 3 is roughly proportional to the number of nuclei that contribute to it, an NMR signal can be used to estimate the number of hydrogen nuclei present in a specimen. Similarly, an MR image can provide an estimate of the distribution of hydrogen nuclei, which are single protons, in a tissue. The number of hydrogen nuclei per unit volume is sometimes called the "proton density", since hydrogen nuclei consist simply of single protons.

A hydrated tissue which is placed in a magnetic field becomes magnetized, and the equilibrium value of its magnetization, M_∞, provides a reasonable estimate of its proton density. The tissue becomes magnetized because its hydrogen nuclei precess about the direction of the applied magnetic field, as shown in Figure 2b. Thus the components of the magnetic moments, in this direction, of all the individual nuclei add together, so that the tissue is magnetized. The precessing nuclei will dissipate their energy by the relaxation processes described in Section II.B. Eventually a state will be reached which is characterized by an equilibrium value of the magnetization, M_∞.

Since most of the hydrogen nuclei in the intervertebral disc are associated with water molecules, M_∞ can be identified with the level of hydration within the tissue. Water accounts for about 80% by weight of healthy nucleus pulposus,[15] and even degenerate annulus fibrosus, where the water content is at its lowest, consists of around 70% by weight of water.[16] Thus, the distribution of M_∞ values within a disc can be used as a measure of the distribution of its water molecules, providing comparable information to the hydration profiles measured by Urban and Maroudas.[17]

M_∞ values are not usually measured on an absolute scale, so that only the relative distribution of water molecules can be inferred. Consequently, results obtained from different images cannot be directly compared, unless the system is calibrated. One possible method of calibration is to enclose a sample of water next to the specimen or person being imaged.[18] However, a similar approach is to compare the distribution of water in a degenerate disc with that in a normal disc which appears in the same image.[19] Although this approach does not yield absolute hydration levels (e.g., in kilograms per cubic meter), it can provide useful information about the differences in hydration across normal and degenerate discs.

D. Formation of an Image

When the magnetic field strength is not uniform, NMR can be used to provide information about the positions of hydrogen nuclei in a sample. According to Equation 1, the Larmor frequency, v_0, depends on the field strength, B_0. Thus, if B_0 is made nonuniform, v_0 will vary with position as will the exact frequency of the RF radiation absorbed.

Figure 4a shows a simple example where the field strength varies linearly from 1.00 to

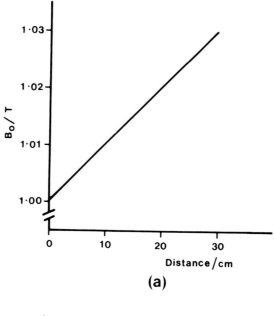

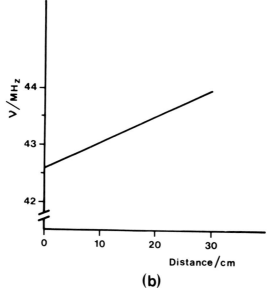

FIGURE 4. The magnetic field gradient in (a) means that the field strength, B_o, is not uniform so that the Larmor frequency, ν_0, varies as shown in (b).

1.03 T over a distance of 30 cm. According to Equation 1, the Larmor frequency then varies linearly from 42.6 MHz at the origin (B_o = 1.00 T) to 43.9 MHz at a distance of 30 cm (B_o = 1.03 T) as shown in Figure 4b. It can also be seen from the graph in Figure 4b that any absorption of RF radiation with a frequency of 43.0 MHz implies the presence of hydrogen nuclei at a distance of 10 cm from the origin. The distribution of B_o values shown in Figure 4a can be arranged by using electromagnets to superimpose a magnetic field gradient of

$$(1.03 - 1.00)/30 = 0.001 \text{ T/cm} \tag{7}$$

on a homogeneous field of 1.00 T.

This simple example shows how, in principle, NMR can be used to provide information about the positions of hydrogen nuclei in a tissue. However, in practice, the techniques used to form an MR image are rather more complicated.

MR images a slice through the body; this slice may represent a sagittal, coronal, or transverse section whose thickness is usually 10 mm but which can be as thin as 5 mm or less. The image consists of discrete, square picture elements, or "pixels". Each individual pixel has a uniform intensity (ranging from white to black) which is called its gray level. Typically several hundred different gray levels are available to be assigned to a pixel to produce contrast in the image. It is difficult to distinguish the individual pixels which make up an image unless there are very few of them. An MR image usually consists of 256 × 256 or 128 × 128 pixels.

The gray level assigned to a pixel depends on the values of M_∞, T_1, and T_2 for the tissue site to which it corresponds. However, the relative contributions of each of these variables to the MR signal, and hence to the gray level of the pixel, depends on the pulse sequence used to record the image (Section II.F).

E. Resolution

The greater the number of pixels in an image, the smaller the structural features which can be observed; MR is unlikely to reliably detect a feature in an object if it is small compared to the distance represented by the size of a pixel. For example, in order to record an MR image of a transverse section of the body, a magnetic field gradient would have to be defined over a distance of about 500 mm. If the image is computed for 128 × 128 pixels, the smallest structural feature which can be detected has dimensions of around

$$500/128 = 4 \text{ mm} \tag{8}$$

However, if the image is computed for 256 × 256 pixels, the smallest detectable feature becomes about

$$500/256 = 2 \text{ mm} \tag{9}$$

in dimension.

The dimension of the smallest object which can be detected is termed the "resolution" of the image. Hence, when the field gradient is defined over 500 mm and the image is divided into 128 × 128 pixels, the resolution is 4 mm. Increasing the number of pixels increases the resolution of the image.

Slice thickness can also affect the assessment of detail in an MR image.[20] It has already been indicated (Section II.D) that the image corresponds to a slice whose thickness is typically 10 mm, but which can be as thin as 1 mm. The thinner the slice, the less the details will be obscured by inhomogeneity of structure throughout its thickness. For example, a 10-mm transverse slice through the midthoracic region must of necessity contain signals from vertebrae as well as from discs — because the discs in this region are only a few millimeters thick.[21] This extraneous signal would tend to degrade the quality of the disc image.

Discs in volunteer subjects have been imaged with a theoretical resolution of 0.8 mm.[20] Figure 5 shows a typical result in which a magnetic field gradient was applied across 200 mm and the image was computed for 256 × 256 pixels. This image corresponds to a slice whose thickness is 5 mm. The laminated structure of the annulus fibrosus cannot be resolved, probably because of slight movements of the body while the image was being recorded (see

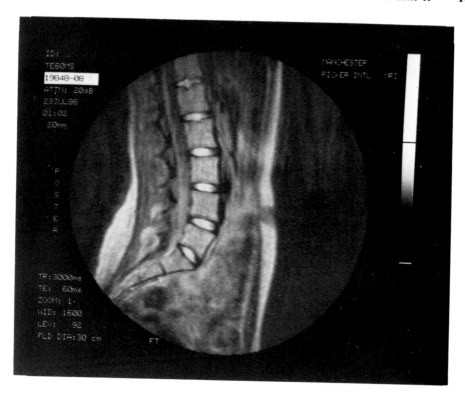

FIGURE 5.   MR image, corresponding to a midline sagittal slice (thickness, 10 mm) through the lumbar region, recorded using an SE30/3000 sequence, from a 22-year-old female, computed for 256 × 256 pixels.

Section II.H). Unfortunately it takes about 25 min to record an image under the conditions used in Figure 5 because of the reduced signal-to-noise ratio when the number of pixels is so large (see Section II.G). Such a long recording time might prove impractical for routine clinical imaging for economic reasons as well as because of the difficulty a patient might experience in staying still for so long (see Section II.H).

Even higher resolution can be attained in images of discs recorded from isolated cadaveric intervertebral joints.[20] The reason is that a magnetic field gradient need then only be applied over a distance of 100 mm. Furthermore, there is no loss of detail associated with movement (Section II.H). Poor signal-to-noise ratios are no longer a serious problem because they can be overcome by imaging for very long periods and by the use of special receiver coils (Section II.G). As a result it has proved possible to record images of cadaveric lumbar discs, like Figure 6, in which the lamellae of the annulus fibrosus can just be resolved, with a theoretical resolution of 0.4 mm. This figure should be compared with Figure 6 of Chapter 1, which is a transverse section subsequently cut from the same disc.

F. Pulse Sequences

In practice, the RF radiation used to record an MR image is not continuous but is pulsed. Figure 7a shows a single pulse which may be represented schematically as shown in Figure 7b. When an RF pulse is applied, the precessing nuclei can absorb energy from it, provided its frequency (represented by the frequency of the sinusoidal oscillations in Figure 7a) corresponds to the Larmor frequency. When the nuclei absorb this energy, they will all precess in unison with the oscillating magnetic field associated with the RF pulse, i.e., they will all precess in phase with each other. As all the nuclei precess in phase, they can induce

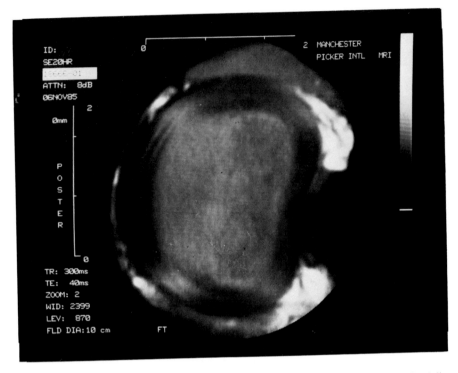

FIGURE 6.   MR image, corresponding to a transverse slice (thickness, 5 mm) through the L3—4 disc of a 16-year-old female cadaveric lumbar spine, recorded using an SE20/300 sequence, computed for 256 × 256 pixels.

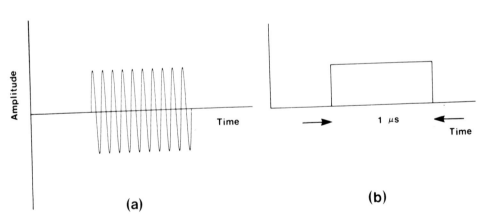

FIGURE 7.   (a) An RF pulse (frequency, 10 MHz) of duration 1 μsec and (b) its schematic representation; the pulses used in MR imaging have a duration of several milliseconds.

an alternating electrical current, whose frequency is equal to their precession frequency, in a receiver coil. However, they gradually dissipate the extra energy, which they have absorbed, by the mechanisms described in Section II.B, and so the relationship between the phases of the precessing nuclei eventually disappears. Consequently, the electrical current in the receiver coil decays. This decay in the induced current, which occurs after the RF pulse, is called the "free induction decay" (FID).

The FID signal is of limited value, and so more complicated sequences of pulses are used; spin-echo (SE) and saturation recovery (SR) sequences have proved especially useful for

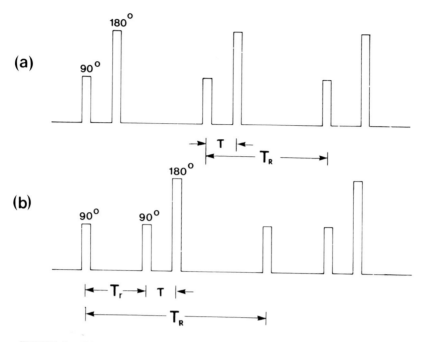

FIGURE 8. Schematic timing diagrams for (a) a spin-echo (SE) sequence (defining the time intervals τ and T_r), and (b) a saturation recovery (SR) sequence (defining the time intervals τ, T_r, and T_R.)

investigating the intervertebral disc.[18] Figure 8a is a schematic timing diagram for the SE sequence which is characterized by a time interval, τ, and a repeat time, T_r. (Some authors use $T_E = 2\tau$ as a measure of the time period.) The current induced in the receiver coil is a measure of the intensity of the NMR signal which, for the SE sequence, is given by

$$S_{SE} = M_\infty \exp(-2\tau/T_2)\{1 - 2\exp(-[T_r - \tau]/T_1) + \exp(-T_r/T_1\} \tag{10}$$

We shall specify an SE sequence by its τ and T_r values, so that an SE20/300 sequence has $\tau = 20$ msec and $T_r = 300$ msec. The SR sequence is characterized by three time intervals, as shown in Figure 8b: the time interval, τ; the repeat time, T_r; and a time interval, T_R, in which the pulse sequence truly repeats. T_R is chosen to be sufficiently long so that FID can occur before the next set of pulses is applied. The intensity of the NMR signal for an SR sequence is then given by

$$S_{SR} = M_\infty \exp(-2\tau/T_2)\{1 - \exp(-T_r/T_1)\} \tag{11}$$

Once again, an SR sequence is specified in the form $SR\tau/T_r$.

By choosing appropriate values of τ and T_r, these pulse sequences can be used to measure T_1, T_2, and M_∞. We shall consider, first of all, measurement of T_1 using SR pulse sequences. Equation 11 can be rewritten in the form

$$\left.\begin{aligned} S_{SR} &= \overline{M}_\infty\{1 - \exp(-T_r/T_1)\} \\ \overline{M}_\infty &= M_\infty \exp(-2\tau/T_2) \end{aligned}\right\} \tag{12}$$

Table 3

**SPIN ECHO (SE) AND SATURATION
RECOVERY (SR) SEQUENCES USED TO
MEASURE THE DISTRIBUTION OF T$_1$ AND T$_2$
VALUES ACROSS THE DISCS OF CADAVERIC
SPECIMENS AND LIVING SUBJECTS**

Cadavers		Living	
T$_1$	T$_2$	T$_1$	T$_2$
SE20/200	SE20/1000	SR12/50	SE20/1000
SE20/300	SE25/1000	SR12/100	SE25/1000
SE20/400	SE30/1000	SR12/150	SE30/1000
SE20/500	SE35/1000	SR12/200	SE35/1000
SE20/760	SE40/1000	SR12/350	SE40/1000
SE20/1000	SE60/1000	SR12/500	SE60/1000
SE20/4000	SE80/1000	SR12/3000	SE80/1000

Note: Sequences are specified by τ/T_r values (see Figure 9) measured in milliseconds.

where $\overline{M}_\infty$ decays slowly during the course of an experiment, and so provides a reasonable estimate of M_∞, provided τ is sufficiently short compared with T_2. If S_{SR} is measured for sufficient values of T_r, with τ fixed at a suitably small value, Equation 12 can be solved to yield M_∞ and T_1. Unfortunately, in some clinical studies, T_1 values have been estimated from only two T_r values; the results are then sensitive to noise (Section II.G) and so may be unreliable. SE sequences can be used to measure T_2. If T_1 is much greater than ($T_r - \tau$), Equation 10 can be written in the form

$$\left. \begin{array}{l} S_{SE} = M_\infty \exp(-2\tau/T_2) \\[2ex] T_1 \gg T_r - \tau \end{array} \right\} \tag{13}$$

By measuring S_{SE} at sufficient values of τ, with T_r fixed at a suitably high value, Equation 13 can be solved to yield M_∞ and T_2. Once again, some clinical estimates of T_2 which rely on only two τ values may be unreliable.

Recently, an iterative method has been developed which yields reliable values for M_∞, T_1, and T_2 from MR images, yet requires data which can be accumulated sufficiently rapidly for clinical investigation.[23] The usual procedure for measuring T_1 by this method is to record MR images using SR sequences with a fixed τ value but different values of T_r. A single image can be calculated from the results in which the gray level of each pixel corresponds to a value of T_1. Thus a map of T_1 values across a slice of tissue is obtained. T_2 values can be calculated from further MR images recorded using SE sequences with a fixed value of T_r but different values of τ. These sequences can be used to calculate a map of T_2 values for a tissue slice. Either the set of SR sequences or the set of SE sequences can be used to compute a map of M_∞ values for the same slice of tissue. Table 3 lists sets of seven sequences which have been used to compute T_1 and T_2, as well as M_∞, maps for both living subjects and cadaveric material by Hickey et al.;[19] note that this iterative procedure allows T_1 to be calculated from SE as well as SR sequences.[23]

Thus, by recording MR images with a range of pulse sequences, an M_∞ map can be computed which provides information on the distribution of water molecules in a slice of intervertebral disc (Section II.C). Similarly, T_1 and T_2 maps provide information on the chemical environment of these water molecules (Section II.D).

G. Noise

As well as the signal induced in the receiver coil, there is also some background noise. This noise can degrade the quality of an MR image in the same way that electrical distrubances (e.g., from the ignition system of a car) can induce signals which interfere with the reception of a radio program. The important factor is how much noise there is compared to the signal to be measured; this is called the signal-to-noise ratio.

Both the slice thickness and the size of the pixels in the image influence the signal-to-noise ratio. If the slice thickness is reduced, there will be fewer nuclei contributing an NMR signal to each pixel in the image. Similarly, increasing the number of pixels, thereby decreasing their size, decreases the number of nuclei which contribute to the signal. In both cases the signal-to-noise ratio will be reduced. For example, if an MR image corresponding to a slice of thickness D is divided into 128×128 pixels, the average signal intensity, $<S>$, per pixel is given by

$$<S> = DAS/(128 \times 128) \tag{14}$$

where S is the average signal emitted by a unit volume of tissue and A is the cross-sectional area of the slice. Now suppose that the slice thickness, D, is halved from 10 mm to 5 mm, while the number of pixels in the image is increased to 256×256. As a result the average signal strength contributing to a pixel becomes

$$<S>' = DAS/(2 \times 256 \times 256) \tag{15}$$

From Equations 14 and 15,

$$<S>' = <S>/8 \tag{16}$$

i.e., the signal intensity per pixel drops by a factor of 8. Since the noise level remains unaffected by changing the slice thickness and the number of pixels, the signal-to-noise ratio must decrease by this same factor and the quality of the image will be impaired.

Thus, there are conflicting criteria for high resolution (see Section II.E) and a high signal-to-noise ratio. It is not surprising that there is a price to be paid for increasing resolution by simply increasing the number of pixels for which the image is computed. The information content of an MR signal from a slice of tissue is determined by physical processes within the slice; it cannot be influenced by subsequent computational procedures. Such procedures (image formation, image analysis, etc.) can present the information in a form which may be easier to understand, but they cannot increase the information content of the signals received.

The signal-to-noise ratio can be improved by averaging several images. For example, Figure 9 compares a single image with averages of two, four, six, and eight such images — all recorded from a single stationary subject with the same SE20/3000 pulse sequence. As the number of images contributing to the average is increased, so the noise level decreases, i.e., the quality of the averaged image is improved. Averaging works because noise arises from random events, whereas NMR signals do not. Different images of the same object will then show different noise patterns which, unlike the features of the image, will tend to cancel out when the images are added. In practice, it is unusual to add images directly, and instead the corresponding NMR signals are averaged. However, the time taken for either process may prove unacceptably long. For example, it took 90 min to record the information used

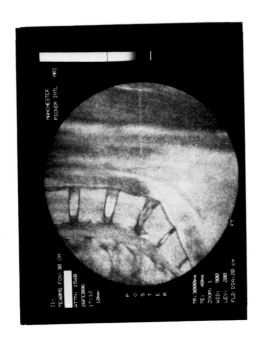

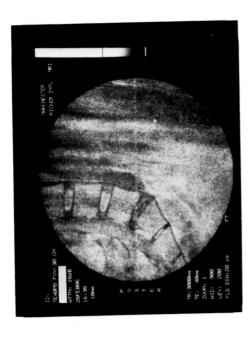

FIGURE 9.   MR image, corresponding to a midline sagittal slice (thickness, 5 mm) through the lumbar region, recorded using an SE20/3000 sequence, from a 39-year-old male with a degenerate L5—S1 disc, represented by 256 × 256 pixels, and obtained by averaging (a) two, (b) four, (c) six, and (d) eight separate images.

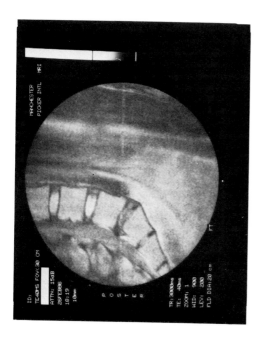

FIGURE 9d

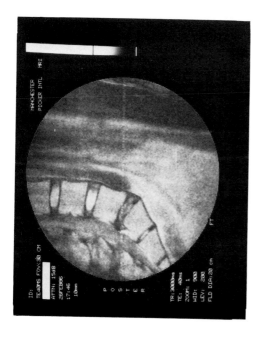

FIGURE 9c

to compute Figure 9d. If the person had moved during this time, the features of the different images would no longer have been in register and the averaging process would have been unreliable (see Section II.H). Furthermore, long imaging times are undesirable in clinical investigations.

The improvement in signal-to-noise ratio is proportional to the square root of the number of images averaged, i.e., four images have to be averaged to double the signal-to-noise ratio. Clearly, if N different MR images are added, the signal contributing to each pixel is increased by a factor of N. However, the random noise can be described by a Poisson distribution,[24] and so increases by only $N^{1/2}$.[25] Therefore, the signal-to-noise ratio increases by $N/N^{1/2} = N^{1/2}$. Consequently, a considerable increase in time is required to obtain much of an improvement. To obtain a tenfold improvement, 100 signals would have to be averaged; if it takes about 6 min to record each image, the subject would have to remain stationary for 10 hr while the necessary signals were being accumulated!

The signal-to-noise ratio can also be improved by using specially designed receiver coils. Conventional receiver coils are an integral part of the MR scanner and surround the body. The signal induced in a coil decreases with increased distance from the precessing nuclear magnets. Thus the signal induced can be increased if a suitable receiver coil is placed very close to the region being imaged. Typically the coil consists of copper tube wound into a helix, like Figure 10a, or a flat coil, like Figure 10b. Helical coils can be used to surround single cadaveric intervertebral joints.[19,20,26] Flat coils are especially useful for obtaining images from selected regions of living people because they can then be placed on the surface of the body, when they are known as surface coils.

Coils are tuned to receive signals with the appropriate Larmor frequency. The natural frequency, v_R, of a coil is given by

$$v_R = 1/2\pi(LC)^{1/2} \tag{17}$$

where L is its self-inductance (measured in henrys) and C is its capacitance (measured in farads). A coil is tuned by adjusting L and/or C until v_R, the frequency at which maximum RF signal is induced, is equal to the Larmor frequency, v_o, of the NMR signal which is to be received. This process is identical to tuning a radio receiver, where it is conventional to vary C (by adjusting a variable capacitor) while L remains fixed. Here L and C depend on the shape and dimensions of the coil. In practice it is conventional to attach a capacitor (typically of a few picofarads capacitance) across its ends. Tuning is achieved either by using a variable capacitor or by systematically changing the shape of the coil.

Our experiments suggest that surface coils will prove more useful for imaging cervical than lumbar discs in vivo. We have obtained images with volunteers lying supine on a surface coil. However, although the posterior regions of the lumbar discs are reasonably close to the coil, their anterior margins are still sufficiently far away that the corresponding regions of the image are comparatively noisy. Because the anterior margins of cervical discs are so much closer to the posterior surface of the neck, surface coils are much more useful for imaging them, as shown in Figure 11.

H. Movement

Movement of a living subject presents a practical problem in recording detailed MR images. Any movement will tend to transfer the NMR signal for one pixel to another and so blur the features of the image, i.e., cause loss of resolution. Furthermore, movement destroys the phase relationships between signals from different parts of the slice and so interferes with the imaging process described in Section III.D. Movement of the spine may be intrinsic, as a result of breathing, or be a result of fidgeting because the person is uncomfortable. Intrinsic movement in the lumbar region is minimized if the person lies

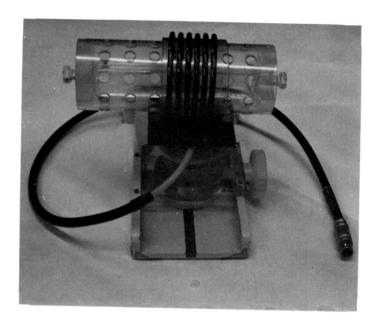

A

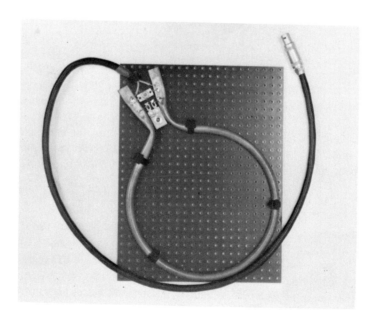

B

FIGURE 10. Copper tube (external diameter, 6 mm) bent into (A) helical and (B) flat receiver coils, for imaging (A) cadaveric specimens and (B) selected regions of living people.

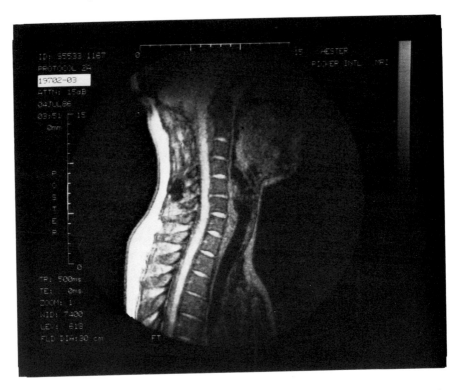

FIGURE 11.   MR image, corresponding to a midline sagittal slice (thickness, 10 mm) through the cervical region, recorded using an FID sequence and surface coil, computed for 256 × 256 pixels.

supine (on the back) rather than prone (on the front). Fidgeting is more of a problem, especially when several images are to be accumulated to improve the signal-to-noise ratio (see Section II.G). People with degenerate discs and who are, therefore, more likely to suffer from back pain, are especially unlikely to be comfortable in an MR scanner for long periods. The effects of movement are a further reason for higher resolution images, with less noise, being obtainable from cadaveric material than from living people.

III. MR IMAGING: FURTHER DETAILS

A. NMR Geometry

In Figure 2a the applied external magnetic field defines a direction which is conventionally labeled as the z axis of a Cartesian coordinate system, as shown in Figure 12. When the nuclear magnet precesses, its magnetization has a component M_z in the z axis direction and a component M_r in the plane perpendicular to it. This component M_r can be resolved into two separate components along the x and y axes which lie in this plane:

$$\left. \begin{aligned} M_x &= M_r \cos\omega_0 t \\ M_y &= M_r \sin\omega_0 t \end{aligned} \right\} \tag{18}$$

where the angular Larmor frequency, ω_0, is defined in Equation 3. It is sometimes convenient to define a Cartesian coordinate system which rotates about the z axis, called the rotating frame, in which the coordinates $\{x', y', z'\}$ are related to those of the Cartesian system $\{x, y, z\}$ by

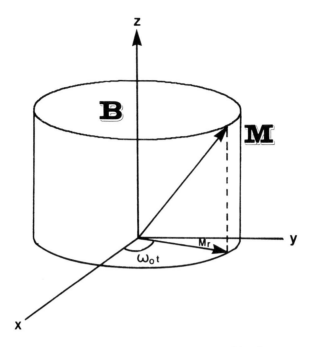

FIGURE 12.   Cartesian coordinate system for describing the precession of a magnetic nucleus, as shown in Figure 2b.

$$\left.\begin{array}{rcl} x' &=& x\cos\omega_0 t \\[1ex] y' &=& y\sin\omega_0 t \\[1ex] z' &=& z \end{array}\right\} \tag{19}$$

In this rotating system the nuclear magnet appears stationary when it precesses in the applied field, B_o, which defines the z axis. Note, however, that the xy and $x'y'$ planes are coincident.

The spin-lattice relaxation time is a measure of the time which the M_z component takes to reach thermal equilibrium with its surroundings. It might seem reasonable to assume that the rate at which M_z increases is proportional to the amount by which it is less than the equilibrium value, M_∞, i.e., that

$$dM_z/dt \; \alpha \; (M_\infty - M_z) = (M_\infty - M_z)/T_1 \tag{20}$$

where Equation 20 acts as a definition of T_1 which is simply a constant of proportionality, for a given system, with the dimensions of time. This equation is one form of the so-called Bloch equations[9] which provide a phenomenological description of NMR.

Rearranging Equation 20 yields

$$\frac{dM_z}{(M_z - M_\infty)} = \frac{-dt}{T_1} \tag{21}$$

which may be integrated with the result

$$\ln(M_z - M_\infty) = -t/T_1 + C \tag{22}$$

where C is a constant of integration, since T_1 is a constant. If we consider a single RF pulse of arbitrary length and a boundary condition of $M_z = M_0$ at $t = 0$, then

$$C = \ln(M_0 - M_\infty) \tag{23}$$

Substituting the expression for C from Equation 23 into Equation 22 yields

$$\frac{M_z - M_\infty}{M_0 - M_\infty} = \frac{-t}{T_1} \Rightarrow M_z = M_\infty + (M_0 - M_\infty)\exp(-t/T_1) \tag{24}$$

This is the mathematical expression describing free induction decay (Section II.F). Thus defining T_1 as a constant of proportionality in a Bloch equation leads to the conclusion that it governs the rate of growth of M_z to its equilibrium value, M_∞, from an initial value M_0.

Similarly, the spin-spin relaxation time is a measure of the time it takes M_r to decay. Although the nuclear magnets precess about the direction of the B_0 field, they only precess in phase when they have absorbed RF radiation (Section II.F). If an RF pulse is applied to produce a transverse component of magnetization, M_r, it seems reasonable to assume that the rate at which this decays will be proportional to the instantaneous magnitude of M_r. The decay of the total M_r for the whole system may then be described by

$$dM_r/dt = -M_r/T_2 \tag{25}$$

which defines T_2 as a constant of proportionality. Rearranging and integrating as before yields

$$\ln M_r = -t/T_2 + K \tag{26}$$

where K is a constant of integration. Applying the boundary condition that when $t = 0$, $M_r = M_1$ allows K to be determined so that Equation 26 becomes

$$\ln(M_R/M_1) = -t/T_2 \Rightarrow M_r = M_1\exp(-t/T_2) \tag{27}$$

Now T_2 can be seen to govern the exponential decay of M_r to zero.

B. Geometry of Pulse Sequences

Because T_1 and T_2 describe decay of magnetization in different directions, the perturbations to the magnetic field which result from the RF pulses of Figure 9 must act in the correct directions if the relaxation times are to be measured. Consider the magnetic nucleus of Figure 2b precessing about the direction of B_0. For an assembly of such nuclei which are not precessing in phase (Section II.F), the resultant magnetization lies along the z axis, and there is no net magnetization in the xy plane. In the rotating frame (Section III.A), the magnetization then acts along z′ as shown in Figure 13a. Now suppose than RF pulse is applied which causes a magnetic field of magnitude B_1 to act along the x′ axis, as shown in Figure 13b. In the coordinate system of Figure 12, B_1 will rotate about z in the xy plane with the Larmor frequency. In order to simplify the description, we return to the rotating frame. Now the magnetization of the assembly of nuclei will start to precess in phase about x′ because they are absorbing energy from the pulse (Section II.F) with a frequency

$$\nu_1 = \gamma B_1/2\pi \tag{28}$$

by analogy with Equation 1. If the pulse is applied for a time t, the magnetization of the sample will tilt through an angle of

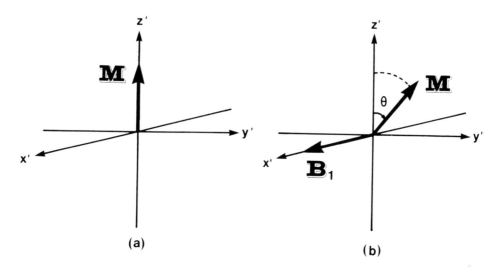

FIGURE 13. The net magnetization, M, of an assembly of magnetic nuclei in a magnetic field B_o, which defines the z' axis of the rotating frame, lines along the z' axis, as shown in (a). However, an RF pulse which applies an additional field, B_1, along x' causes M to rotate toward y' by an angle, θ, as shown in (b).

$$\theta = 2\pi\nu_1 t = \gamma B_1 t \tag{29}$$

toward the y' axis, as shown in Figure 13b. By adjusting B_1 or t, the tilt angle can be controlled. Typically the magnetization is rotated through 90° (from along z' to along y'), which is called a 90° pulse, or though 180° (from along z' to $-z'$) by a 180° pulse.

We shall use the SE sequence of Figure 8a to explain how pulse geometry is exploited in the measurement of relaxation times. In this sequence[27] a 90° pulse shifts the net magnetization of the sample from along z' to along y', as shown in Figures 14a and b. However, if there are slight inhomogeneities in B_o, the individual nuclei experience slightly different fields and so precess with slightly different frequencies in the coordinate system of Figure 12. Thus, after some more time has elapsed, the individual nuclei will have slightly different directions for their magnetization, as shown in Figure 14c, and so the net magnetization in the x'y' plane is decreased. Consider the direction OA, corresponding to the highest precession frequency (i.e., moving clockwise away from y' when viewed down z'), and the direction OB, corresponding to the lowest (i.e., moving anticlockwise from y'). Suppose a 180° pulse is applied when a time interval τ has elapsed after the initial 90° pulse. OA is rotated to OA' and OB to OB', as shown in Figure 14d. Since OA' and OB' are moving in the same direction as before, they will now tend to come together after a further time interval of τ has elapsed, i.e., an echo occurs at time 2τ after the 90° pulse. The same argument can be applied to all the nuclei so that the magnitude of the magnetization would be restored, after a time interval 2τ, to that when the 90° pulse was first applied.

However, the magnitude of the magnetization decreases because of relaxation processes. In the SE sequence the magnetization is confined to the x'y' (i.e., the xy) plane. Thus in time 2τ, the magnetization will decrease by a factor of $\exp(-2\tau/T_2)$ (Section III.A). By measuring the signal induced in the receiver coil, the decrease in magnetization at times 0 and 2τ can be detected and T_2 calculated. In practice the procedure is repeated several times, as indicated in Figure 8a, to obtain a better estimate of T_2. A variation of the technique called the Carr-Purcell sequence,[28] involves following the 180° pulse by a series of further 180° pulses, with a time interval 2τ, and observing the decay in the sample magnetization.

C. Slice Selection

Selection of a slice to be imaged perpendicular to the z axis involves addition of a field

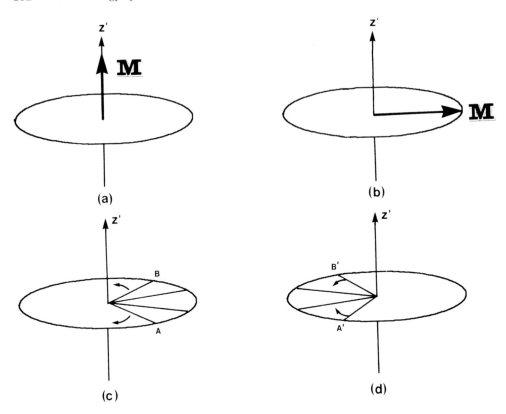

FIGURE 14.   (a) Before the first pulse of the spin-echo (SE) sequence, shown in Figure 8a, is applied, the net magnetization of an assembly of magnetic nuclei lies along z', as in Figure 13a. (b) When a 90° pulse is applied, the magnetization is rotated into the x'y' plane. (c) After some time has elapsed the individual nuclei dephase so that their individual magnetization directions are different; for example, OA and OB are then moving apart, in the directions shown, in the rotating frame. (d) At a time interval τ a 180° pulse rotates the directions of magnetization so that OA rotates to OA' and OB to OB'; since OA' moves in the same direction as OA, and OB' moves in the same direction as OB, they are now moving toward each other as shown.

gradient to B_o, as shown in Figure 15. Now Equation 1 will only be satisfied, i.e., RF radiation with $v = v_o$ will only be absorbed in the plane defined by $z = z_o$. However, we have seen in Section II.B that RF waves with v values close to v_o can also be absorbed — although not as efficiently. Since absorption can occur over a range of frequencies, Δv (see Figure 3), NMR signals can be obtained over a range, Δz, of z values centered at z_o. The steeper the applied gradient, the smaller Δv will be, i.e., the thinner the slice which can be imaged. It is not simple to predict the slice profile because it depends on the RF pulse sequence, which is applied repeatedly, and the shape of the individual pulses; computer simulation of the imaging process is usually necessary for the prediction.[29,30]

D. Two-Dimensional Imaging

Once a slice has been selected, as described in Section III.C, its image can be obtained. The method described here was introduced by Kumar et al.,[31,32] which, as indicated by Mansfield and Morris,[13] is simply related to the two-dimensional Fourier transform techniques used in NMR spectroscopy. It is worth noting that this was not the approach adopted initially for MR imaging;[5,6] a number of methods have been described by Mansfield and Morris.[13]

At an initial time t = 0, an RF pulse rotates the magnetization of the nuclei into the xy (i.e., the x'y') plane. Magnetic field gradients are then superimposed on B_o at defined times along the x and y directions so that the total field at some position in the slice is given by

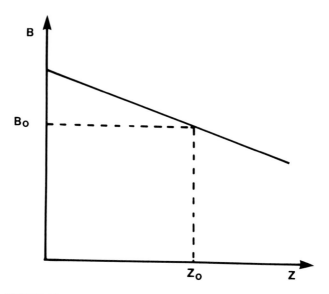

FIGURE 15. The field gradient in the z axis direction means that RF radiation of frequency $\nu = \nu_o$ will only be absorbed when the field strength $B = B_o$, i.e., in the plane defined by $z = z_o$.

$$B(x, y) = \begin{cases} B_0 + g_x(t)x & 0 < t \leq t_x \\ B_0 + g_y(t)y & t > t_x \end{cases} \tag{30}$$

where $g_x(t)$ is a linear gradient applied in the x direction in the period t_x and $g_y(t)$ is a linear gradient applied in the y direction. Now the Larmor frequency depends on position in the field $B(x,y)$ and is given, from Equation 1, by

$$\begin{aligned} \nu(x, 0) &= \gamma(B_0 + g_x(t)x)/2\pi & t \leq t_x \\ \nu(0, y) &= \gamma(B_0 + g_y(t)y)/2\pi & t > t_x \end{aligned} \tag{31}$$

Since the Larmor frequency depends on position, so does the phase of the NMR signal induced in the receiver coil. According to Equation 31 the phase then depends on the x coordinate at time $t \leq t_x$ and on the y coordinate with $t > t_x$ and is given by

$$\begin{aligned} \varphi(x) &= 2\pi\nu(x, 0)t_x & t = t_x \\ \varphi(y) &= 2\pi\nu(0, y)(t - t_x) & t > t_x \\ &= 2\pi\nu(0, y)t_y \end{aligned} \tag{32}$$

From Equations 31 and 32,

$$\left.\begin{array}{ll}\varphi(x) = \gamma[B_0 + g_x(t)x]t_x & t = t_x \\ \varphi(y) = \gamma[B_0 + g_y(t)y]t_y & t > t_x \end{array}\right\} \tag{33}$$

Consider the NMR signal from an elemental area dxdy. Its magnitude is proportional to the number of protons, which depends on the proton density per unit area of the slice, $M(x,y)$ (Section II.C). However, the signal is subject to T_2 decay (Section III.A). Its phase is given by Equation 33 and so depends on t_x and t_y for a given set of gradients. The NMR signal can thus be represented both in amplitude and phase by

$$ds(t_x, t_y) \propto M(x, y)dxdy \exp(-t/T_2) \exp i[\varphi(x) + \varphi(y)] \tag{34}$$

If we now put

$$m(x, y) = M(x, y)\exp(-t/T_2) \tag{35}$$

then the signal $S(t_x, t_y)$ from the total slice is given by

$$S(t_x, t_y) = \int_{x=-\infty}^{\infty} \int_{y=-\infty}^{\infty} m(x,y)\exp i[\varphi(x) + \varphi(y)]dxdy \tag{36}$$

by integrating Equation 34 and ignoring a constant of proportionality. $S(t_x,t_y)$, the signal from the entire slice a time t after application of the original RF pulse, can then be seen to be the two-dimensional Fourier transform of $m(x,y)$. According to the inversion property of Fourier transforms (see, for example, References 33 and 34),

$$m(x, y) = \int_{t_x=0}^{\infty} \int_{t_y=0}^{\infty} S(t_x, t_y)\exp[-i(\varphi(x) + \varphi(y))]dt_x dt_y \tag{37}$$

since $S(t_x,t_y) = 0$ for t_x and $t_y < 0$ and neglecting a factor of $(2\pi)^2$.

Thus if the experimental procedure is repeated with sufficient values of t_x and t_y, the integral of Equation 37 can be solved numerically. As a result $m(x,y)$ is recovered, i.e., an image of the slice is obtained which in this example depends on the proton density and T_2.

E. Chemical Shifts

Equation 1 has to be modified slightly when the atoms containing the magnetic nuclei are bonded to other atoms in molecules; however, this complication only becomes apparent when the magnetic field, B_0, is relatively high (above 1 T). Since the electrons in an atom or molecule are charged and in motion, their paths will be influenced by B_0. As a result, an induced field, $\sigma_s B_0$ is set up to oppose the applied field, where σ_s is a constant for a given arrangement of electrons. Consequently the Larmor frequency is reduced to

$$\nu_s = \gamma B_0(1 - \sigma_s)/2\pi \tag{38}$$

by analogy with Equation 1. Thus ν_o is shifted from its expected value by an amount which, in a molecule, depends on the chemical bonding around the magnetic nucleus.

In order to define the chemical shift it is necessary to have a reference compound. For hydrogen nuclei the reference is invariably tetramethylsilane, $Si(CH_3)_4$, abbreviated to TMS; in this compound the 12 hydrogen nuclei are all equivalent, and we may express their Larmor frequency, ν_R, by

Table 4
CHEMICAL SHIFT, δ, FOR
THE HYDROGEN NUCLEI
IN VARIOUS MOLECULES

Molecule	δ
Saturated hydrocarbons[a]	1
Water	4.76
Aromatic hydrocarbons	7

[a] Most of the hydrogen nuclei in fats
are in a saturated hydrocarbon
environment.

$$\nu_R = \gamma B_0 (1 - \sigma_R)/2\pi \qquad (39)$$

as in Equation 38. The chemical shift is then defined, empirically, by

$$\delta = 10^6 (\nu_s - \nu_R)/\nu_R \qquad (40)$$

which can be related to the constants σ_s and σ_R (sometimes referred to as "shielding constants") by

$$\left. \begin{aligned} \delta &= 10^6 (\sigma_R - \sigma_s)/(1 - \sigma_R) \\ &\simeq 10^6 (\sigma_R - \sigma_s) \quad \sigma_R \ll 1 \end{aligned} \right\} \qquad (41)$$

from Equations 38, 39, and 40. Values of δ for hydrogen nuclei in different chemical environments are listed in Table 4.

At the lower fields which are commonly used in MR imaging systems ($B_0 \sim 0.2$ T) chemical shifts are negligible; however, at higher fields ($B_0 \sim 2$ T) used in some imaging systems the effect is appreciable.[25,36] The Larmor frequency for hydrogen nuclei in water is different from that for hydrogen nuclei in fats. Consequently, regions of high field images which correspond to parts of the tissue with a high fat content will be out of register with those regions corresponding to high water content. Images show chemical shift artifacts unless they are then corrected numerically for this effect.

However, chemical shifts have the advantage that they can be used to determine the chemical environment of magnetic nuclei. Indeed a molecule which contains magnetic nuclei has a characteristic NMR spectrum. This spectrum consists of signal strength plotted against ν; peaks are displaced from the value of ν_0 for the type of nucleus being investigated by an amount which depends on chemical shift effects.[37] High values of B_0 and a uniformity of 1 part in 10^7 are required to resolve the peaks of the spectrum. (Resolution of the peaks in a spectrum should not be confused with the spatial resolution of an MR image.) In imaging systems with sufficiently high magnetic fields, MR images can be used to identify regions of interest from which spectra are to be recorded. A spectrum can then be recorded from this region by defining a volume from which NMR signals are to be detected in much the same way as slices are selected for imaging (Section III.C).[38]

Changes in chemical shifts which arise from ^{31}P atoms changing their chemical environments during metabolic reactions have proved highly informative.[39] Generally these experiments involve purely spectroscopic techniques and do not make use of MR images. Although

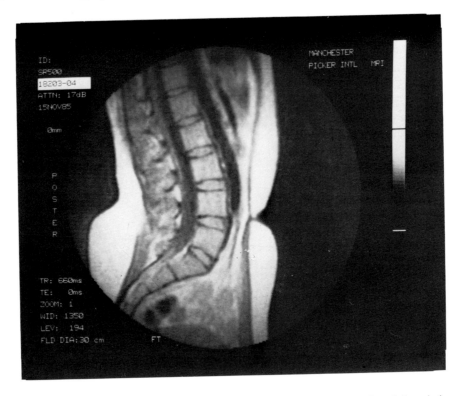

FIGURE 16.   MR image, corresponding to a midline sagittal slice (thickness, 10 mm) through the lumbar region, recorded using an SR12/500 sequence, from a 19-year-old in which the annulus and nucleus cannot be distinguished.

this kind of approach has yet to be applied to the intervertebral disc, it may prove possible to compare metabolic levels in normal and degenerate discs from ^{31}P chemical shifts.

F. Contrast Media

One advantage of MR imaging over X-ray techniques, including CT, is that contrast media are not needed to image or characterize soft tissues. Nevertheless, paramagnetic ions (e.g., Cu^{2+}, Fe^{3+}, and Gd^{3+}) have sufficient effect on T_1 that their introduction into biological systems, in order to enhance contrast in MR images, has been proposed. For example, gadolinium compounds containing the Gd^{3+} ion have been introduced into small blood vessels to make them easier to see in MR images.[40-43] However, there are no applications of paramagnetic ions to imaging the intervertebral disc yet reported in the literature.

IV. INVESTIGATION OF THE DISC

A. T$_1$- and T$_2$-Weighted Images

The appearance of the intervertebral disc in an MR image depends on the pulse sequence used. For example, the annulus and nucleus can be clearly distinguished in all the discs appearing in Figure 5, which was recorded with an SE30/3000 sequence. However, in Figure 16, which was recorded with an SR12/500 sequence, there is little contrast between annulus and nucleus. It is not surprising that the contrast is not the same in the two images because the signal strength depends on M_∞, T_1, and T_2 (Section II.D) and the relative contribution of each depends on the pulse sequence (Section II.F).

Images recorded using pulse sequences which are especially sensitive to T_2 (known as T$_2$-weighted images) provide excellent contrast between annulus and nucleus. SE sequences with long τ and T_r values, like the SE30/3000 sequences used to obtain Figure 5, are very sensitive to T_2 (Section II.F) and so provide T_2-weighted images. Because they allow the annulus and nucleus to be so clearly distinguished, they are commonly used in qualitative MR imaging studies of the disc.[1,2]

Annulus and nucleus are difficult to distinguish in images which are recorded with pulse sequences which are more sensitive to T_1 values and are, therefore, said to be T_1-weighted. SE sequences with short τ and T_r values and SR sequences with short τ values provide T_1-weighted images like Figure 16 where there is little contrast between nucleus and annulus.

The reason why SE sequences with low τ and T_r values are T_1-weighted can be illustrated by manipulation of Equation 10; this paragraph presents the derivation and may be skipped without loss of continuity. Note that

$$\exp(x) \simeq 1 + x \qquad x \ll 1 \tag{42}$$

Given the values of T_1 and T_2 for a healthy nucleus pulposus (Section II.B), if we assume that $\tau \ll T_2$ and T_r is chosen such that $T_r \ll T_1$ and $T_r \gg \tau$, Equation 10 can then be approximated by

$$\begin{aligned}
S_{SE} &= M_\infty \{1 - 2\tau/T_2\}\{1 - 2[1 - (T_r/T_1) + (\tau/T_1)] + [1 - (T_r/T_1)]\} \\
&= M_\infty \{1 - 2\tau/T_2\}\{(T_r - 2\tau)/T_1\} \\
&\simeq M_\infty (T_r/T_1) \tag{43}
\end{aligned}$$

Equation 43 illustrates that, under these conditions, the strength of the NMR signal is sensitive to T_1 but is insensitive to T_2. A similar analysis may be performed for SR sequences with short τ values like the SR12/500 sequence used to record Figure 16.

Experiments on cadaveric discs allow the information which can be obtained from MR images recorded with different pulse sequences to be compared directly with anatomical observation.[19,20,44] For example, high-resolution MR images of cadaveric discs have been recorded using suitable gradients and the special receiver coil (Section II.G) shown in Figure 10a.[19] In these experiments the best definition of annulus and nucleus was obtained with an SE20/4000 sequence which showed little structure within the annulus.[20] Reduced contrast between annulus and nucleus occurred with an SE20/300 sequence which did, however, demonstrate the laminated structure of the annulus, as shown in Figure 6. Comparison of this image with a transverse section subsequently cut from the same disc showed that the MR image represented true structural features (Section II.E). Examination of cadaveric material using an SE25/300 sequence also allowed the more collagenous outer lamellae to be distinguished from the inner annulus and nucleus of the disc.[44] This observation is consistent with the view that the inner and outer lamellae of the annulus have slightly different functions which are reflected in their chemical composition (see also Chapter 1, Section V).[45] These considerations may prove useful for investigation of disc degeneration using cadaveric material. However, we have already seen that such high-resolution images are unlikely to be attained in clinical images (Section II.E) because of patient movement (Section II.H). Thus T_2-weighted images are likely to be employed for routine clinical investigation of disc pathology.

B. Qualitative Studies

Because soft tissues can be distinguished without the use of contrast media, herniated discs can be identified in MR images, and narrowing of the disc space can be easily seen.[1,2,46-52] Edelman et al.[53] have claimed that MR is as useful for detecting protrusions as either computed tomography or myelography. A posterior bulge of the L5—S1 disc can be

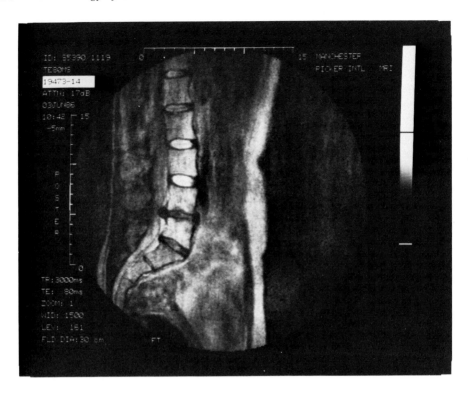

FIGURE 17.   MR image, corresponding to a midline sagittal slice (thickness, 10 mm) through the lumbar region, recorded using an SE40/3000 sequence, showing posterior protrusion of the disc at the L4—5 level. (Courtesy of Dr. J. P. R. Jenkins, Department of Diagnostic Radiology, University of Manchester, England, 1986.)

seen in Figure 9d, and a more obvious example of a herniated disc appears in Figure 17. Protrusion of nucleus into the cancellous bone of the L3 and L4 vertebral bodies can also be seen in the MR image of Figure 18.

Loss of the signal intensity from the nucleus in T_2-weighted images provides clear evidence of disc degeneration.[2,46-52,54] In Figure 9d, recorded with an SE20/3000 sequence, the nucleus and annulus can be distinguished for all the discs except L5—S1 where the signal from the nucleus is remarkably low. Since this sequence yields T_2-weighted images (Section IV.A), the reduction in signal from the nucleus of this disc presumably arises from a reduced T_2 value. A similar decreased signal intensity, from the nucleus of certain discs, is apparent in Figures 17 (L4—5 and L5—S1) and 18 (L5—S1). Many reports have identified this decrease in signal with degeneration,[14,46-52,54] although a similar effect occurs as a result of aging.[50] Nevertheless, a single disc with a reduced signal from the nucleus in a T_2-weighted image, where the annulus and nucleus of the other discs can be readily distinguished, is presumably degenerate. Such discs often show posterior protrusions as in Figure 17. Furthermore, in our experience of investigating volunteer subjects (aged less than 40 years), lumbar discs with reduced signal from the nucleus in T_2-weighted images only occur in people who have suffered from back pain.

It is not clear from the literature whether MR imaging can detect calcification of the disc. Paushter et al. imply that it cannot because there is no signal from calcified sites.[1] Edelman et al. agree that, as expected, MR images are far less sensitive to calcification than the results of computed tomography.[53] However, they believe that calcification of herniated nucleus is indicated by regions of decreased signal intensity in both T_1- and T_2-weighted images.[53] Calcification of the disc arises from deposition of calcium pyrophosphate dihydrate,

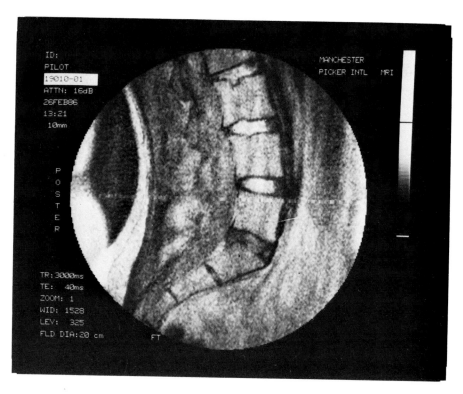

FIGURE 18. MR image, corresponding to a midline sagittal slice (thickness, 5 mm) through the lumbar region, recorded using an SE20/3000 sequence, from a 26-year-old female showing degenerate discs at the L5—S1 level as well as protrusion of the nucleus into vertebrae.

$Ca_2P_2O_7 \cdot 2H_2O$, or hydroxyapatite, $Ca_5(PO_4)_3OH$.[55] Solids have shorter T_2 values than liquids[11] which would lead to reduction of intensity in a T_2-weighted image. Whether this effect is detectable as a result of disc calcification is uncertain as fibrous collagenous tissues can also have very low T_2 values.

MR imaging is more reliable than the conventional technique of discography for diagnosis of disc degeneration.[56] In discography, contrast medium is injected into the nucleus of discs in sedated patients under local anesthetic; degeneration is indicated by leakage of contrast medium through fissures.[57] We have already seen that degeneration is also indicated by loss of signal from the nucleus in T_2-weighted MR images. Gibson et al. examined 22 patients and graded 50 of their discs on a scale of 0 (healthy) to 4 (grossly degenerate) using both discography and MR.[56] Their results are summarized in Figure 19, which shows that the two techniques agree remarkably well; indeed, there was no discrepancy at all for grades 3 and 4, where it would be most important to detect degeneration. Six discrepancies occurred. In three cases degeneration was initially overlooked in the discograms but was apparent in the MR images; in a further two discography was unsuccessful because of incorrect needle placement.[56] MR only failed to detect one degenerate disc identified by discography. Sometimes clefts appear in discograms of the nucleus; it has been claimed that they also appear in T_2-weighted MR images.[58] However, studies on cadaveric material show that the apparent cleft in MR images does not represent any obvious anatomical feature.[44] Nevertheless, MR has proved to be a very reliable technique for identifying discs by the decreased signal from the nucleus in T_2-weighted images.

C. Quantitative Studies

T_1 and T_2 values for the nucleus both decrease during aging, but T_1 is more reliable than

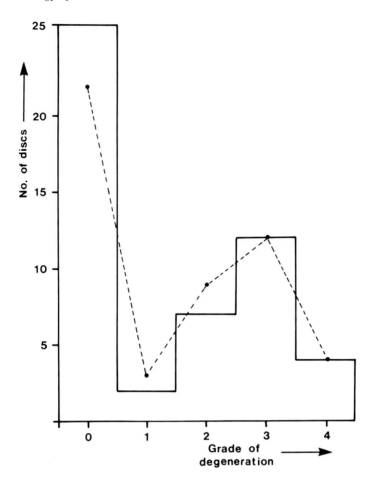

FIGURE 19. Comparison of the assessment of disc degeneration by MR imaging and discography. Fifty discs were examined and graded on scale of 0 (healthy) to 4 (grossly degenerate) by the two techniques.[56] The continuous line shows the distribution of grades allocated by discography, and the dashed line represents allocation by MR imaging.

T_2 for detecting degeneration. Of course, it would be difficult to use T_1-weighted images to determine whether discs were degenerate because of the lack of contrast between nucleus and annulus demonstrated by Figure 16. Calculation of T_1 values, as described in Section II.F, overcomes this problem and provides a quantitative technique for identifying degenerate discs. Such calculations also provide values of M_∞, which are a measure of water content in discs (Section II.C).

Values of T_1 and T_2 have been calculated for the nuclei of both normal and degenerate discs in living subjects and in segments of lumbar spine dissected from cadavers.[14,18,19,59] Jenkins et al. showed that the average T_1 value for the nucleus, and its average T_2 value, both decreased with age, as shown in Figure 20, for discs which appeared normal in T_2-weighted images of patients.[14] However, Figure 20a indicates that T_1 values are consistently lower for the nuclei of degenerate discs; indeed, an analysis of their results showed that T_1 values for the nuclei of surgically proven degenerate discs were significantly lower ($p < 0.01$) than normal values, even in the older age groups.[14] Figure 20b indicates that decreased values of T_2 are less reliable for detecting degeneration because they are not very different from normal values for the nuclei of older discs; the average value of T_2 for the nuclei of degenerate discs is not significantly different ($p > 0.05$) from its value for normal discs in

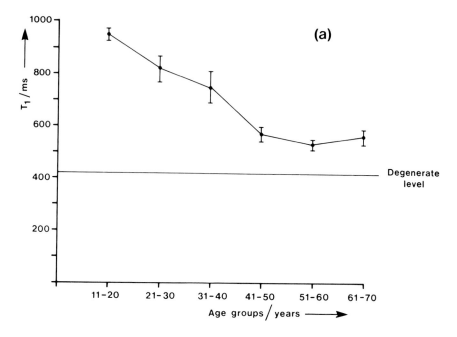

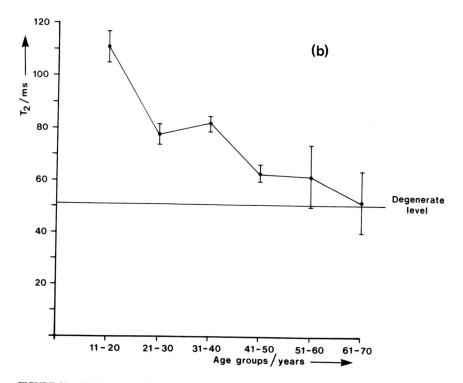

FIGURE 20.   Values of (a) T_1 and (b) T_2 for the nucleus of normal discs in age ranges from 11 to 20 to 61 to 70 years compared with the corresponding value for degenerate discs.[14] Error bars represent the standard error of the mean.

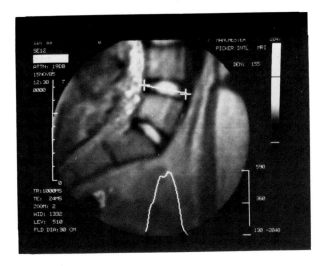

FIGURE 21.   Map of M_∞ values for the lumbar region of a 21-year-old female with no degenerate discs, computed from MR images corresponding to a sagittal slice (thickness, 5 mm). Values of M_∞ across the bisector of the L4—5 disc (marked) are superimposed on the figure.

the age range 61 to 70 years.[14] Furó et al. showed that both T_1 and T_2 values were correlated with the water content of cadaveric discs.[59] Since dehydration of the disc is associated with aging and degeneration (see Section II.B of Chapter 1), they suggested that T_1 as well as T_2 values could be used to detect degeneration, as has indeed proved to be feasible.[14]

MR images can also be used to determine the distribution of M_∞, T_1, and T_2 values for discs in vivo in order to provide further information on aging and degenerative changes.[18,19] Figure 17 of Chapter 1 corresponds to a map of M_∞ values within a transverse slice of the L3—4 disc in a segment of the lumbar spine of a 16-year-old cadaver. Although this figure cannot provide absolute values for the water content (in kilograms per cubic meter), because the experiment was not calibrated (see Section II.C), the gray level of each pixel is proportional to the hydration level of the volume of the disc to which it corresponds. The densitometer trace across the anterior-posterior axis, which is superimposed on this figure, shows that the high water content of the nucleus gradually decreases throughout the thickness of the annulus to its lowest value on the periphery of the disc; this distribution of M_∞ values is consistent with the hydration profiles determined by direct measurement of water content is selected portions of discs from young cadavers.[17] Analysis of MR images from the L3—4 disc of a 82-year-old cadaver indicated a very different distribution of water, in which the water content of the nucleus was comparable to that of the annulus, once again in accordance with expectation (see Volume I, Chapter 1, Section II.C) and with direct measurement of hydration profiles.[17] Similar differences occur in the distribution of T_1 and T_2 values. In the younger disc the relaxation times had highest values in the nucleus which gradually decreased through the inner annulus to their lowest values in the outer annulus; in the older disc the distribution of relaxation times was much more uniform.[19] Since M_∞ is a measure of water content (Section II.C), while relaxation times provide information on the environment of these water molecules (Section II.B), it appears that the chemical environment of the water molecules changes during age-related dehydration of the disc.

Results from living subjects are comparable to those from cadaveric material; the main difference is that calculations have been performed on sagittal slices because of the difficulty of selecting true transverse slices of the discs of living people.[18,19] Figure 21 corresponds to a map of M_∞ values calculated for a sagittal section of lumbar spine with no degenerate discs; a graph of M_∞ values along the bisector of the L4—5 discs is superimposed on this figure and shows a similar distribution of water to that obtained in vitro (Volume I, Chapter 1, Figure 17). Normal and degenerate discs may be identified in a T_2-weighted image. However, subsequent investigation may involve comparison of M_∞, T_1, and T_2 values. Figure 22c compares the distribution of M_∞ values along the bisectors of normal and degenerate discs in the same patient; in this example the L3—4 disc was normal, while the L4—5 level was degenerate. The degenerate disc clearly has a dehydrated nucleus when compared with normal. Furthermore, Figures 22a and 22b clearly show a reduction in the T_1 and T_2 values for the nucleus of the degenerate disc, as compared with the results from the normal disc, as well as showing how these values are distributed.

It is clear that aging and degeneration are associated with a change in the chemical environment of the water molecules in the nucleus, as well as simply with dehydration. The correlation between reduced relaxation times and water loss may arise simply because the average environment of a water molecule changes when the proportion of water, relative to organic matter, decreases. Alternatively, the decrease in relaxation times may indicate specific biochemical changes which occur during aging, perhaps, for example, a change in the relative proportions of water associated with collagen and proteoglycans. In either case these results are consistent with the view that degeneration represents an extreme form of aging changes, with T_1 values as the most sensitive indicator of degeneration.

IV. CONCLUSIONS

MR imaging provides a noninvasive technique for examining living discs which is free from the hazards associated with ionizing radiation. A further advantage is that soft tissues can be seen and distinguished from each other without using contrast media. So far no risks associated with either magnetic fields or the levels of RF radiation involved have been identified. The only exception is that some patients cannot be examined because the magnetic field reacts adversely with pacemakers, steel clips, artificial heart valves, etc. Any ferromagnetic material, i.e., one which contains metallic iron, nickel, or cobalt and their alloys (but not chemical compounds containing them), will experience appreciable forces in the magnetic field; thus the positions and proper functioning of any devices containing such materials will be greatly disturbed with the risk of considerable trauma. Although consideration of possible hazards has tended to concentrate on the effects of magnetic fields on biological systems, it would appear that dissipation of the energy supplied to the tissues by the RF pulses provides a more likely source of potential risk. This energy raises the energy of the magnetic nuclei (the ^1H nuclei when imaging the intervertebral disc), as described in Section II.A, and is then dissipated by spin-lattice and spin-spin interactions (Section II.B); eventually this energy will be dissipated as heat to the surrounding tissues. However, if the heating effect is not too great, the temperature of the tissues may be controlled by normal homeostatic mechanisms, and for vascular tissues blood flow will reduce any local heating effects. No such problems have yet been identified at the levels of RF energy associated with this technique.

As a result of its advantages, MR imaging provides a valuable clinical technique for identifying degenerate discs and examining their structures. A degenerate disc can be readily identified by the low signal from the nucleus, in a T_2-weighted image (Section III.A), which makes its demarcation from the annulus virtually impossible. Thus a degenerate disc has a distinctive appearance when compared with the other discs in a T_2-weighted image of the spine, as exemplified by the appearance of the L5—S1 disc in Figure 9d. Posterior protrusion of the disc, which might be associated with entrapment of nerve roots, can be easily seen (Figure 17), as can protrusion of the nucleus into the cancellous bone of the vertebral bodies (Figure 18). Analysis of images obtained with a suitable range of RF pulse sequences (Table

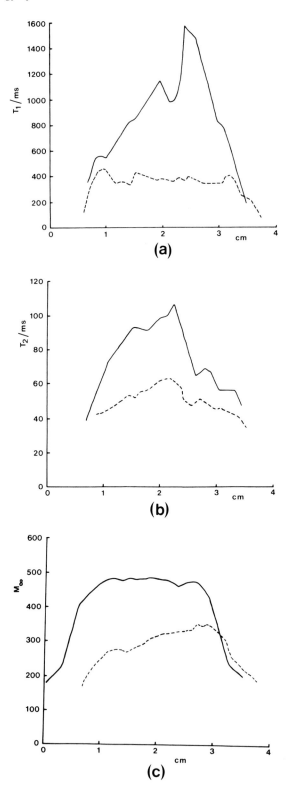

FIGURE 22.   A comparison of the distribution of (a) T_1, (b) T_2, and (c) M_∞ values along the bisectors of a normal L3—4 (continuous line) and a degenerate L4—5 (dashed line) in the spine of the same 23-year-old. These results were computed from MR images corresponding to a sagittal slice (thickness, 5 mm). (Courtesy of Dr. J. P. R. Jenkins, Department of Diagnostic Radiology, University of Manchester, England,1976.)

3) provides a quantitative indication of degeneration. However, the time required to obtain the necessary images may prove unacceptable either because the patient cannot stay still for long enough or because there is insufficient time available on the scanner for such a detailed investigation of a single patient. The major disadvantage of MR imaging for routine assessment of disc pathology and in clinical research is its high cost. This disadvantage is probably more of a problem in the U.K. than in other advanced countries where a greater proportion of financial resources is available for health care and clinical research.

MR imaging is a valuable research technique because it provides information on the distribution of water and its chemical environment in the disc, as well as showing gross structure; furthermore, it can provide this information for the discs of living patients and volunteer subjects, as well as for cadaveric material. Determination of the relative hydration of the various parts of the disc is important because it is the swelling pressure exerted by water that allows the disc to withstand compressive load (see Volume I, Chapter 1, Section II.A). MR images can provide this information on the discs of living people, allowing hydration to be related to pathology. Relaxation times are sensitive to the chemical environment of the water molecules. While this chemical environment may well prove to be related to the water content, the two kinds of information are quite distinct in principle. MR images are thus sensitive to the detailed biochemistry of the disc and allow biochemical information to be obtained from pathological discs in living people. The technique of MR imaging is already proving valuable. It has many further potential applications for basic research into the etiology of disc degeneration as well as for providing a sensitive assessment and imaging technique for clinical research.

ACKNOWLEDGMENTS

We thank Professor I. Isherwood for the provision of facilities for MR imaging and for encouragement and Dr. J. P. R. Jenkins for allowing us to use images obtained in his clinical research. We are also grateful to Karen Davies for preparing the illustrations, to Pat Mellor and Peggy Burt for typing, and to Celia Hukins for help with the literature. R. M. A. and D. S. H. are supported by grants from the Medical Research Council.

REFERENCES

1. **Paushter, D. M., Modic, M. T., and Masaryk, T. H.,** Magnetic resonance imaging of the spine: applications and limitations, *Rad. Clin. North Am.,* 23, 551, 1985.
2. **Richardson, M. L., Genant, H. K., Helms, C. A., Gillespy, T., Heller, M., Jergesson, H. E., and Bovill, E. G.,** Magnetic resonance imaging of the musculoskeletal system, *Orthop. Clin. North Am.,* 16, 569, 1985.
3. **Bloch, F., Hansen, W. W., and Packard, M. E.,** Nuclear induction, *Phys. Rev.,* 69, 127, 1946.
4. **Purcell, E. M., Torrey, H. C., and Pound, R. V.,** Resonance absorption by nuclear magnetic moments in a solid, *Phys. Rev.,* 69, 37, 1946.
5. **Lauterbur, P. C.,** Image formation by induced local interactions: examples employing nuclear magnetic resonance, *Nature (London),* 242, 190, 1973.
6. **Mansfield, P. and Grannell, P. K.,** NMR "diffraction" in solids, *J. Phys. C,* 6, L422, 1973.
7. **Gabillard, R.,** Mesure du temps de relaxation T_2 en présence d'une inhomogénéité de champ magnétique supérieure à la largeur de raie, *C. R. Acad. Sci. (Paris),* 232, 1551, 1951.
8. **Gabillard, R.,** Theory and measurement of relaxation times in nuclear paramagnetic resonance, *Rev. Sci., (Paris),* 90, 307, 1952.
9. **Abragam, A.,** *The Principles of Nuclear Magnetism,* Clarendon Press, Oxford, 1961.
10. **Andrew, E. R.,** *Nuclear Magnetic Resonance,* Cambridge University Press, Cambridge, England, 1958.
11. **Farrar, T. C. and Becker, E. D.,** *Pulse and Fourier Transform NMR: Introduction to Theory and Methods,* Academic Press, London, 1971.

12. **Gadian, D. G.,** *Nuclear Magnetic Resonance and Its Application to Living Systems,* Clarendon Press, Oxford, 1982.

13. **Mansfield, P. and Morris, P. G.,** *NMR Imaging in Biomedicine,* Academic Press, New York, 1982.

14. **Jenkins, J. P. R., Hickey, D. S., Zhu, X. P., Machin, M., and Isherwood, I.,** MR imaging of the intervertebral disc: a quantitative study, *Br. J. Radiol.,* 58, 705, 1985.

15. **Gower, W. E. and Pedrini, V.,** Age-related variations in the protein-polysaccharides from human nucleus pulposus, annulus fibrosus and costal cartilage, *J. Bone Jt. Surg.,* 51-A, 1154, 1969.

16. **Stevens, R. L., Ryvar, R., Robertson, W. R., O'Brien, J. P., and Beard, H. K.,** Biologic changes in the annulus fibrosus in patients with low back pain, *Spine,* 7, 223, 1982.

17. **Urban, J. P. G. and Maroudas, A.,** Measurement of fixed charge density in the intervertebral disc, *Biochim. Biophys. Acta,* 586, 166, 1979.

18. **Hickey, D. S.,** Quantitative magnetic resonance studies of normal and degenerate discs, in *Back Pain: Methods for Clinical Investigation and Assessment,* Hukins, D. W. L. and Mulholland, R. C., Eds., Manchester University Press, Manchester, England, 1986, 91.

19. **Hickey, D. S., Aspden, R. M., Hukins, D. W. L., Jenkins, J. P. R., and Isherwood, I.,** Analysis of magnetic resonance images from normal and degenerate lumbar intervertebral discs, *Spine,* 11, 702, 1986.

20. **Hickey, D. S., Aspden, R. M., and Hukins, D. W. L.,** High resolution magnetic resonance imaging of the intervertebral disc, in *Back Pain: Methods for Clinical Investigation and Assessment,* Hukins, D. W. L. and Mulholland, R. C., Eds., Manchester University Press, Manchester, England, 1986, 118.

21. **Pooni, J. S., Hukins, D. W. L., Harris, P. F., Hilton, R. C., and Davies, K. E.,** Comparisons of the structure of human intervertebral discs in the cervical, thoracic and lumbar regions of the spine, *Surg. Radiol. Anat.,* 8, 175, 1986.

22. **McDonald, G. G. and Leigh, J. S.,** A new method for measuring longitudinal relaxation times, *J. Magn. Reson.,* 9, 358, 1973.

23. **Hickey, D. S., Checkley, D., Aspden, R. M., Naughton, A., Jenkins, J. P. R., and Isherwood, I.,** A method for the clinical measurement of relaxation times in magnetic resonance imaging, *Br. J. Radiol.,* 59, 565, 1986.

24. **Moroney, M. J.,** *Facts from Figures,* Penguin, Harmondsworth, England, 1951.

25. **Braddick, H. J. J.,** *The Physics of Experimental Methods,* 2nd ed., Chapman & Hall, London, 1963.

26. **Hoult, D. I., and Lauterbur, P. C.,** The sensitivity of the zeugmatographic experiment involving human samples, *J. Magn. Reson.,* 34, 425, 1979.

27. **Hahn, E. L.,** Spin echoes, *Phys. Rev.,* 80, 580, 1950.

28. **Carr, H. Y. and Purcell, E. M.,** Effects of diffusion on free precession in nuclear magnetic resonance experiments, *Phys. Rev.,* 94, 630, 1954.

29. **Locher, P. R.,** Computer simulation of selective excitation in NMR imaging, *Philos. Trans. R. Soc. London, Ser. B.,* 289, 537, 1980.

30. **Robinson, E., Hickey, D. S., and Aspden, R. M.,** Computer simulation of slice profile effects in magnetic resonance imaging of the spine, in *Back Pain: Methods for Clinical Investigations and Assessment,* Hukins, D. W. L. and Mulholland, R. C., Eds., Manchester University Press, Manchester, England, 1986, 128.

31. **Kumar, A., Welti, D., and Ernst, R. R.,** Imaging of macroscopic objects by NMR Fourier zeugmatography, *Naturwissenschaften,* 62, 34, 1975.

32. **Kumar, A., Welti, D., and Ernst, R. R.,** NMR Fourier zeugmatography, *J. Magn. Reson.,* 18, 69, 1975.

33. **Bracewell, R.,** *The Fourier Transform and Its Applications,* McGraw-Hill, London, 1965.

34. **Champeney, D. C.,** *Fourier Transforms and Their Physical Applications,* Academic Press, London, 1973.

35. **Soila, V. P., Viamonte, M., and Starewicz, P. M.,** Chemical shift misregistration effects in MR imaging, *Radiology,* 153, 819, 1984.

36. **Dwyer, A. J., Krop, R. H., and Hoult, D. I.,** Frequency shift artifacts in MR imaging, *J. Comput. Assisted Tomography,* 9, 16, 1985.

37. **Lynden-Bell, R. M. and Harris, R. K.,** *Nuclear Magnetic Resonance Spectroscopy,* Nelson, London, 1969.

38. **Bottomley, P. A., Foster, T. B., and Darrow, R. D.,** Depth-resolved surface-coil spectroscopy (DRESS) for *in vivo* ^1H, ^{31}P and ^{13}C NMR, *J. Magn. Reson.,* 59, 338, 1984.

39. **Radda, G. K.,** Control of bioenergetics: from cells to man by phosphorus nuclear magnetic resonance spectroscopy, *Biochem. Soc. Trans.,* 14, 517, 1986.

40. **Runge, V. M., Clanton, J. A., Lukehart, C. M., Partain, C. L., and James, A. E.,** Paramagnetic agents for contrast-enhanced NMR imaging; a review, *Am. J. Roentgenol.,* 141, 1209, 1983.

41. **Weinmann, H.-J., Brasch, R. C., Press, W. R., and Wesbey, G. E.,** Characteristics of gadolinium-DTPA complex: a potential NMR contrast agent, *Am. J. Roentgenol.,* 142, 619, 1984.

42. **Runge, V. M., Clanton, J. A., Foster, M. A., Smith, F. W., Lukehart, C. M., Jones, M. M., Partain, C. L., and James, A. E.,** Paramagnetic NMR contrast agents: development and application, *Invest. Radiol.,* 19, 408, 1984.

43. **Runge, V. M., Schoerner, W., Niendorf, H. P., Laniado, M., Koehler, D., Claussen, C., Felix, R., and James, A. E.,** Initial clinical evaluation of gadolinium DTPA for contrast-enhanced magnetic resonance imaging, *Magn. Reson. Imaging,* 3, 27, 1985.

44. **Pech, P. and Haughton, V. M.,** Lumbar intervertebral disc: correlative MR and anatomic study, *Radiology,* 156, 699, 1985.

45. **Klein, J. A. and Hukins, D. W. L.,** Functional differentiation in the spinal column, *Eng. Med.,* 12, 83, 1983.

46. **Chafetz, N. T., Genant, H. K., Moon, K. L., Helms, C. A., and Morris, J. M.,** Recognition of lumbar disc herniation with NMR, *Am. J. Roentgenol.,* 141, 1153, 1983.

47. **Han, J. S., Kaufman, B., El Yousef, S. J., Benson, J. E., Bonstelle, C. T., Alfidi, R. J., Haaga, J. R., Yeung, H., and Huss, R. G.,** NMR imaging of the spine, *Am. J. Roentgenol.,* 141, 1137, 1983.

48. **Modic, M. T., Weinstein, M. A., Paulicek, W., Starnes, D. L., Duchesneau, P. M., Boumphrey, F., and Hardy, R. J.,** Nuclear magnetic resonance imaging of the spine, *Radiology,* 141, 757, 1983.

49. **Modic, M. T., Weinstein, M. A., Paulicek, W., Boumphrey, F., Starnes, D., and Duchesneau, P. M.,** Magnetic resonance of the cervical spine: technical and clinical observations, *Am. J. Roentgenol.,* 141, 1129, 1983.

50. **Modic, M. T., Paulicek, W., Weinstein, M. A., Boumphrey, F., Ngo, F., Hardy, R., and Duchesneau, P. M.,** Magnetic resonance imaging of intervertebral disk disease, *Radiology,* 152, 103, 1984.

51. **Modic, M. T. and Weinstein, M. A.,** Nuclear magnetic resonance of the spine, *Br. Med. Bull.,* 40, 183, 1984.

52. **Crawshaw, C., Kean, D. M., and Mulholland, R. C.,** The use of nuclear magnetic resonance in the diagnosis of lateral canal entrapment, *J. Bone Jt. Surg.,* 66-B, 711, 1984.

53. **Edelman, R. R., Shoukimas, G. M., Stark, D. D., Davis, K. R., New, P. J. F., Saini, S., Rosenthal, D. I., Wismer, G. L., and Brady, T. J.,** High-resolution surface-coil imaging of lumbar disk disease, *Am. J. Roentgenol.,* 6, 479, 1985.

54. **Norman, D., Mills, C. M., Brant-Zawadzki, M., Yeates, A., Crooks, L. E., and Kaufman, L.,** Magnetic resonance imaging of the spinal cord and canal: potentials and limitations, *Am. J. Roentgenol.,* 141, 1147, 1983.

55. **Ball, J.,** New knowledge of intervertebral disc disease, *J. Clin. Pathol.,* 31 (Suppl. Royal College of Pathologists 1), 200, 1978.

56. **Gibson, M. J., Buckley, J., Mawhinney, R., Mulholland, R. C., and Worthington, B. S.,** Magnetic resonance imaging and discography in the diagnosis of disc degeneration, *J. Bone Jt. Surg.,* 68-B, 369, 1986.

57. **McCulloch, J. A. and Waddell, G.,** Lateral lumbar discography, *Br. J. Radiol.,* 51, 498, 1978.

58. **Aguila, L. A., Piranaino, D. W., Modic, M. T., Dudley, A. W., Duchesneau, P. M., and Weinstein, M. A.,** The internuclear cleft of the intervertebral disc: magnetic resonance imaging, *Radiology,* 155, 155, 1985.

59. **Furó, I., Bobert, M., Pócick, and Tompa, K.,** *In vitro* ¹H NMR "mapping" of human intervertebral discs, *Magn. Reson. Imaging Med.,* 3, 146, 1986.

INDEX